Human Well-Being Research and Policy Making

This series creates a dialogue between well-being scholars and well-being public policy makers.

Well-being theory, research and practice are essentially interdisciplinary in nature and embrace contributions from all disciplines within the social sciences. With the exception of leading economists, the policy relevant contributions of social scientists are widely scattered and lack the coherence and integration needed to more effectively inform the actions of policy makers.

Contributions in the series focus on one more of the following four aspects of well-being and public policy:

- Discussions of the public policy and well-being focused on particular nations and worldwide regions
- Discussions of the public policy and well-being in specialized sectors of policy making such as health, education, work, social welfare, housing, transportation, use of leisure time
- Discussions of public policy and well-being associated with particular population groups such as women, children and youth, the aged, persons with disabilities and vulnerable populations
- Special topics in well-being and public policy such as technology and well-being, terrorism and well-being, infrastructure and well-being.

More information about this series at http://www.springer.com/series/15692

el-Sayed el-Aswad

The Quality of Life and Policy Issues among the Middle East and North African Countries

Springer

el-Sayed el-Aswad
Independent Scholar
Bloomfield Hills, MI, USA

ISSN 2522-5367 ISSN 2522-5375 (electronic)
Human Well-Being Research and Policy Making
ISBN 978-3-030-00325-8 ISBN 978-3-030-00326-5 (eBook)
https://doi.org/10.1007/978-3-030-00326-5

Library of Congress Control Number: 2018954621

This Springer imprint is published by the registered company Springer Nature Switzerland AG
The registered company address is: Gewerbestrasse 11, 6330 Cham, Switzerland

This book is dedicated to the people of the Middle East and North Africa region, people living at the grassroots in this region, and to those in the region who are fighting to enhance their quality of life, happiness, and well-being.

Preface

The Middle East and North Africa region, including the Gulf States (hereafter the MENA region), is made up of countries that have received considerable attention by scholars and the media, especially since the terrorist events of September 11, 2001 directed at the United States (el-Aswad 2013), the financial crisis of 2008 that resulted in a sharp downturn in the economies of financially advanced countries, the Arab Spring of 2011 that impacted the political and social well-being of people throughout the MENA region (el-Aswad 2016), and the current and ongoing wars being fought in Syria and Yemen with their profoundly negative impact on the well-being of people in the predominately Islamic countries of North Africa and West Asia.

The book, first of the Springer book series of Human Well-Being Research and Policy Making, is a timely work in that it addresses quality of life in the 21 nations of the Middle East and North Africa Region by focusing on multiple policy dimensions of well-being, including economy, health, education, technology, and social welfare among other objective as well as subjective dimensions of quality of life and well-being. The study deals with culturally, socioeconomically, demographically, and politically diverse countries that make up the MENA region. By broadly addressing the social realities that characterize the MENA countries, the research reported in this monograph seeks to delineate cross-cultural similarities and differences by extensively and comparatively focusing on six of the region's most influential countries—Egypt, Iran, Israel, Turkey, Tunisia, and the United Arab Emirates (UAE), selected specifically to highlight the diversity found in the region.

This monograph reflects a holistic approach to the analysis of a wide range of policy frameworks that currently are in place in the MENA region. The monograph also identifies the major *drivers* of governmental and private sector approaches to well-being policy development that impact directly on the quality of life of the more than 381 million people living in the region—approximately 6% of the world's total population. The approach to policy development analysis adopted in this monograph is intended to both advance our understanding of the nature of well-being policy development under the conditions of the considerable political turbulence that exists in the region and, at the same time, suggests with broad brush strokes the dimensions of a more coherent policy framework designed to enhance the quality of life of the people that are living in a defined geographic area and are loosely joined together through a shared faith—in this case, predominately Islam and its teachings (Estes and Tiliouine 2016; Tiliouine and Estes 2016).

Further, the policy analysis approach adopted in the monograph assigns priority to the enhanced well-being of people and their development as the central focus of policy development in the region and its neighbors more broadly. Thus, and as viewed from the author's perspective,

> At the center of well-being is a deep sense of peace, personal satisfaction, and happiness within ourselves and in our relationships with others. All four of these states of being—peace, personal satisfaction, happiness, and well-being—are outcomes achieved through a combination of personal reflection and interpersonal exchanges. They also are associated with the often-complex interplay of the social, political, economic, religious, ideological, and other forces that surround us (Estes 2017: 3).

This monograph demonstrates the special appeal and significance of such interrelated topics as quality of life, well-being, and policy issues.

About the Book

The book contains six chapters: Chap. 1, *Introduction* and Chap. 2, *Methodology* present the main approach, which is to address well-being and policy issues from multiple lenses. Chapter 3, *Historical Background*, delineates briefly and in broad terms the successes, challenges, quality of life, and overall human development experienced by the MENA region from ancient to present times. This chapter provides a rationale for identifying 21 countries as comprising the MENA region as well as for focusing on 6 selected countries, Egypt, Iran, Israel, Tunisia, Turkey, and the UAE, for the purpose of extensive comparative inquiries. In addition, the chapter provides an account of the region's core geographic, demographic, and political features as well as its overall human development achievements, particularly in the domains of economy, health, and education. Other key characteristics of the MENA region in terms of culture, religion, ideology, minority relationships, technological developments, and militarization are provided. Within this historical context, the chapter addresses external and internal factors along with religious and ideological orientations impacting the quality of life in the MENA region.

Chapter 4, *Indicators of Quality Of Life and Well-Being in the MENA Region: A Comparative Analysis*, focuses on the quality of life and well-being issues in the selected MENA countries (Egypt, Iran, Israel, Tunisia, Turkey, and the UAE). This chapter applies multiple objective and subjective indicators to assess multiple dimensions of well-being including health, education, economy, work force, communication, technology, human rights, happiness, religious freedom, tolerance, political terror, corruption, and freedom of expression, to mention a few. This chapter presents a comparative analysis focusing on indicators of equity and inequality in differing domains of human development and well-being or ill-being. In addition, the chapter concludes that despite the variations in quality of life across the MENA region, there is a cross-cultural similarity or a common pattern of well-being related mainly to the progress made in the multiple dimensions of people's lives. In brief, although indicators of freedom of expression, religious tolerance, and happiness are still low in the MENA countries, they have achieved remarkable progress in overall human development, particularly in the domains of health care, education, economy, and technology.

Chapter 5, *Key Drivers of Well-being and Policy Issues in the MENA Region*, investigates the staging of drivers of well-being and social–public policies in the MENA region. The essential thesis or objective of this inquiry is to show to what extent the drivers, indicators, and outcomes of well-being help the policy makers generate sociocultural plans and public policies aimed at improving the quality of life of people living in the MENA region. This study provides an assessment of the relative role of economic and noneconomic drivers such as health, education, economy, demography, political stability, security, technology, and culture in shaping policy priorities and the policy options available to the MENA region. The chapter addresses the most critical challenging factors hindering social–public policies from improving the quality of life in the MENA region. This research underscores that, although the ordinary people in the MENA region work diligently to improve their standards of living, the major challenges facing them relate mostly to incapacitated governments and inept political systems. The chapter, however, proposes that a better understanding of the drivers and determinants of well-being in the MENA region will provide relevant considerations concerning policy issues in that region.

Chapter 6, *Conclusion*s, provides the most important findings of the research and recommendations to authorities and policy makers interested in the promotion of well-being and quality of life in the MENA countries. Put simply, this chapter accentuates the fact that well-being research can help policy makers target public services in effective manners and guide national and regional authorities in implementing social policies adequately and productively toward advancing people's lives.

Bloomfield Hills, USA el-Sayed el-Aswad

References

el-Aswad, el-S. (2013). Images of Muslims in Western scholarship and media after 9/11. *Digest of Middle East Studies,* 22 (1), 39–56.

el-Aswad, el-S. (2016). State, Nation and Islamism in contemporary Egypt: An anthropological perspective. *Urban Anthropology,* 45 (1–2), 63–92.

Estes, R. J. (2017). The search for well-being: From ancient to modern times. In R. J. Estes & M. J. Sirgy (Eds.), *The Pursuit of Human Well-Being: The Untold Global History* (pp. 3–30). Dordrecht, NL: Springer.

Estes, R. J., & Tiliouine, H. (2016). Social development trends in the Fertile Crescent region: Jordan, Iraq, Lebanon and Syria. In H. Tiliouine & R. J. Estes (Eds.), *The state of social progress of Islamic societies: Social, economic, political, and ideological challenges* (pp. 179–210). Cham, Switzerland: Springer International Publishing.

Tiliouine, H., & Estes, R. J. (2016) Social development in North African countries: Achievements and current challenges. In H. Tiliouine & R. J. Estes (Eds.), *The State of social progress of Islamic societies: Social, economic, political, and ideological challenges* (pp. 109–136). Cham, Switzerland: Springer International Publishing.

Acknowledgements

Serving tenure at universities in the United States, Egypt, Bahrain, and the United Arab Emirates has given me the opportunity to advance cross-cultural perspectives that I used in this study. I hope the reader finds reading this book as enriching an experience as I have had through investigating patterns of quality of life and well-being of the people of the Middle East and North Africa.

This book would not have been written without the invitation, endorsement, and inspiration of Richard J. Estes and M. Joseph Sirgy, editors of the Springer book series of *Human Well-Being Research and Policy Making*. The comments and feedback of Richard J. Estes and M. Joseph Sirgy as well as of anonymous peer viewers and scholars have enriched and deepened the scholarly discussion of the book.

I would like to thank David Walker for preparing the graphics and figures to underscore the complicated and multidimensional data of the research. Many thanks go to Pamela Fried for providing careful copy editing of the book.

I also thank my family for the great support and unique ways in which they contributed during the production of this monograph. My wife, Mariam, provided editorial assistance. My son, Kareem, helped me prepare a portion of the statistics. My son, Amir, aided in fashioning the map of the MENA region by using *Adobe Photoshop* and *Adobe Illustrator*.

I am grateful to the editorial team at Springer International Publisher with special thanks to Esther Otten, Eric Schmitt, Thomas Hempfling, Hendrikje Tuerlings, Almitra Ghosh, and Prashanth Ravichandran for their administrative assistance for this work.

Bloomfield Hills, Michigan
July 2018

With appreciation,
el-Sayed el-Aswad

Contents

About the Author

Prof. el-Sayed el-Aswad, Ph.D. received his doctorate in anthropology from the University of Michigan, Ann Arbor. He has taught at Wayne State University (USA), Tanta University (Egypt), Bahrain University, and United Arab Emirates University (UAEU). He achieved the CHSS-UAEU Award for excellence in scientific research publication for the 2013–2014 academic year. He served as Chairperson of the Sociology Departments at both the UAEU and Tanta University as well as the Editor in Chief of the *Journal of Horizons in Humanities and Social Sciences: An International Refereed Journal* (UAEU). He has published widely in both Arabic and English and is the author of *Muslim Worldviews and Everyday Lives* (AltaMira Press, 2012), *Religion and Folk Cosmology: Scenarios of the Visible and Invisible in Rural Egypt* (Praeger Press, 2002; translated into Arabic in 2005) and *The Folk House: An Anthropological Study of Folk Architecture and Traditional Culture of the Emirates Society* (*al-Bait al-Sha'bi*) (UAE University Press, 1996).

He has been awarded fellowships from various institutes including the Fulbright Program, the Ford Foundation, the Egyptian government, and the United Arab Emirates University. He is a member of Editorial Advisory Boards of the *Digest of Middle East Studies (DOMES)*, Muslims in Global Societies Series, Tabsir: *Insight on Islam and the Middle East,* and *CyberOrient* (Online Journal of the Middle). He is a member of the American Anthropological Association, the Middle Eastern Studies of North America, the American Academy of Religion, and the International Advisory Council of the World Congress for Middle Eastern Studies (WOCMES). He has published eight books, over eighty papers in peer-reviewed and indexed journals, and over 30 book reviews.

Abbreviations and Acronyms

DIAC	Dubai International Academic City
DKV	Dubai Knowledge Village
FGH	Financing Global Health
FH	Freedom House
GCC	Gulf Co-operation Council
GDP	Gross domestic product
GFP	Global Firepower Index
GMI	Global Militarization Index
HAAD	Health Authority Abu Dhabi
ICT	Information and Communications Technology
IHME	Institute for Health Metrics and Evaluation
ILO	International Labor Organization
ILS	Internet Live Stats
IMF	International Monetary Fund
IT	Information technology
IWS	Internet World Stats
MENA	Middle East and North Africa
NGO	Non-governmental organization
OECD	Organization for Economic Cooperation and Development
OPEC	Organization of the Petroleum Exporting Countries
PPP	Purchasing Power Parity; Public–Private Partnership
SDGs	United Nations' Sustainable Development Goals
SGI	Sustainable Governance Indicators
SPI	Social Progress Index
UN	United Nations
UNDAF	United Nations Development Assistance Framework
UNDP	United Nation Development Programme
UNESCO	United Nations Educational, Scientific, Cultural Organization
UNHCR	United Nations High Commissioner for Refugees
UNICEF	United Nations Children's Fund

UNRISD	United Nations Research Institute for Social
WB	World Bank
WDA	World Data Atlas
WEF	World Economic Forum
WFP	World Food Programme
WHO	World Health Organization

List of Figures

List of Tables

Chapter 1
Introduction

Abstract This chapter provides a brief review of scholarly literature examining quality of life and well-being policy, globally and regionally. It also addresses core objectives and key questions related to well-being and policy issues in the MENA region.

Keywords Quality of life · Well-being · Social-public policy
Human development

Quality of life indicates "well-being" as well as the entire scale of human experiences, states, perceptions, and domains of thought concerning standards of "the good life." It also involves judgments of the value placed on the experiences of communities regarding satisfaction with life across typical aspects of daily living such as health, income, education, work, family, and leisure (Massam 2002; Peter and Machin 2015; Theofilou 2013). This monograph identifies important indicators and measurements of progress in people's economic, health, and educational development as a whole. It also investigates the systems of social and public policies implemented in the MENA region impacting economic, health, and educational well-being.

Well-being policy is *welfarist* in the sense that it presumes that well-being and the creation of opportunities for the pursuit of happiness should be among the concerns of policy makers (Haybron and Tiberius 2015; Helliwell et al. 2016). Research on regional well-being can assist policy makers in directing their efforts toward identifying the most effective policies that reap positive outcomes that lead people toward better lives. In this context, the concepts of well-being and welfare are used here interchangeably. Academic researchers as well as policy makers engaged in analyzing and promoting well-being and quality of life in the Middle East and North Africa (MENA) region are likely to appreciate this work. In addition, this book would be suitable not only for use in university classrooms (undergraduate and graduate levels) but also in seminar activities. It is most likely that scholars and teachers of the world and Middle East studies would choose the book for their courses because it deals with contemporary MENA countries from cross-cultural perspectives. It is expected that local, national, and regional authorities in the MENA region can use information

el-S. el-Aswad, *The Quality of Life and Policy Issues among the Middle East and North African Countries*, Human Well-Being Research and Policy Making,
https://doi.org/10.1007/978-3-030-00326-5_1

regarding the drivers and indicators of well-being from the findings of this study as an integrating guide to their future plans and actions in the field of public services.

For over four decades the scholarly literature addressing quality of life and well-being worldwide has been extensive (Brixi et al. 2015; Diener 1984; Diener et al. 2003; Diener et al. 2010; Estes 1993, 2007, 2010, 2012, 2015; Estes and Sirgy 2017; Estes et al. 2017; Galloway 2006; Glatzer et al. 2015; Huppert and Cooper 2014; Kwon 2005; Lammy and Tyler 2014; McGillivray and Clarke 2007; Michalos 2004, 2014; Oishi 2010; Roy 2010; Sirgy 1998, 2011; Sirgy et al. 2017). In addition to the significant contributions to the scholarship of development and well-being in the MENA region (el-Aswad 2017; Estes and Tiliouine 2014; Jawad 2015; Karshenas and Moghadam 2006, 2009; Moghadam and Karshenas 2006; Silva et al. 2012; Tiliouine and Estes 2016; Tiliouine and Meziane 2017), this monograph presents new grounds for cross-cultural inquiries regarding quality of life and policy issues among countries of that region.

This book examines the roles of state institutions, international development agencies, religious and sectarian-based community services, non-governmental organizations and private sectors in improving the quality of life in the respective countries being studied. The research uses indicators and data from economic, health, and education among other resources, including the *Human Development Index*, to capture both positive and negative states of the quality of life in the MENA region. In other words, finance, health, and education are considered to be among the most important aggregate measures in the assessment of well-being. With regard to economic well-being, the study addresses economic recourses and living standards by comparing the gross domestic product per capita of different counties (United Nations Development Programme 2016). Concerning health well-being, the study relies on and compares key health indicators such as life expectancy at birth, occurrences of diseases, and incidences of infant and maternal mortality rates among countries. Regarding educational well-being, the inquiry uses indicators such as expected years of schooling, adult literacy, and gross enrollment in basic, secondary, and tertiary school levels.

This book provides policy analysts and decision makers with otherwise hard to obtain data and information concerning a wide array of development experiences needed to identify policy issues and outcomes at the local, regional, national, and international levels. The objectives of the monograph can be summarized as follows:

1. To present a critical review of the scope of the changing quality of life in MENA countries with respect to economic, health, and educational and, where appropriate, technological and environmental well-being.
2. To examine the systems of social and public policies implemented in the MENA countries impacting economic, health, and educational well-being.
3. To analyze the positive and negative aspects of well-being policy enacted in the MENA region in terms of the three dimensions.

This monograph is critical to understanding the place MENA countries now occupy in the world. It identifies significant drivers of human well-being of the people in the MENA region. The book explores the interrelationships among the transition outcomes (i.e., economic, health, and educational progress) and the many drivers or factors influencing such outcomes—socioeconomic, cultural, demographic, technological, institutional, and political factors.

Specifically, this book seeks to answer the following questions:

What is the historical context of the quality of life and policy issues among the MENA countries?

What are the present circumstances concerning the quality of life and policy issues within the MENA region?

What are the core indicators of quality of life and well-being in the MENA region?

What are the major drivers of human well-being successes in the MENA countries being studied?

To what extent do social and public policies improve the quality of life among the people of the MENA countries?

What are the practical goals and lessons that can be achieved from contemporary practices of policy issues in the MENA region?

What types of additional policy initiatives are needed to bring peace and harmony to the region and, thus, open new pathways for attaining progressively higher levels of well-being for all the countries in the MENA region?

References

Brixi, H., Ellen, L., & Woolcock, M. (2015). *Trust, voice, and incentives*. Washington DC: World Bank Publications.

Diener, E. (1984). Subjective well-being. *Psychological Bulletin, 95*(3), 542–575.

Diener, E., Oishi, S., & Lucas, R. E. (2003). Personality, culture, and subjective well-being: Emotional and cognitive evaluations of life. *Annual Review of Psychology, 54,* 403–425.

Diener, E., Kahneman, D., & Helliwell, J. (2010). *International differences in well-being*. Oxford UK: Oxford University Press.

el-Aswad, el-S. (2017). *Well-being in the Arab world: An anthropological perspective.* Paper presented at the International Conference on Social and Related Sciences, 4–8 Oct. Side-Antalya, Turkey.

Estes, R. J. (1993). Toward sustainable development: From theory to praxis. *Social Development Issues, 15*(3), 1–29.

Estes, R. J. (2007). *Advancing quality of life in a turbulent world*. Dordrecht: Springer.

Estes, R. J. (2010). The world social situation: Development challenges at the outset of a new century. *Social Indicators Research, 98,* 363–402.

Estes, R. J. (2012). Economies in transition: Continuing challenges to quality of life. In K. Land, A. C. Michalos, & M. J. Sirgy (Eds.), *Handbook of social indicators and quality of life research* (pp. 433–457). Dordrecht: Springer.

Estes, R. J. (2015). Global change and quality of life indicators. In F. Maggino (Ed.), *A life devoted to quality of life* (pp. 173–193). Dordrecht: Springer.

Estes, R. J., & Sirgy, M. J. (2017). *The pursuit of human well-being: The untold global history.* Dordrecht: Springer.

Estes, R. J., & Tiliouine, H. (2014). Islamic development trends: From collective wishes to concerted actions. *Social Indicators Research, 116,* 67–114.
Estes, R. J., et al. (2017). Well-being in Canada and the United States. In R. J. Estes & M. J. Sirgy (Eds.), *The pursuit of human well-being* (pp. 257–299). Dordrecht: Springer.
Galloway, S. (2006). Quality of life and well-being: Measuring the benefits of culture and sport: Literature review. *Scottish Executive Social Research, 12,* 3–93.
Glatzer, W., et al. (2015). *Global handbook of well-being and quality of life.* New York: Springer.
Haybron, D., & Tiberius, V. (2015). Well-being policy: What standard of well-being? *Journal of the American Philosophical Association, 1*(4), 712–733.
Helliwell, J., Huang, H., & Wang, S. (2016). *World Happiness Report 2016, Update* (Vol. I). New York: Sustainable Development Solutions Network. Retrieved from https://s3.amazonaws.com/happiness-report/2016/HR-V1Ch2_web.pdf.
Huppert, F. A., & Cooper, C. L. (2014). *Interventions and policies to enhance wellbeing: A complete reference guide* (Vol. VI). Chichester: Wiley.
Jawad, R. (2015). *Social protection and social policy systems in the MENA region: Emerging trends.* New York: United Nations Department of Economic and Social Affairs. http://www.un.org/esa/socdev/csocd/2016/RJawad-MENA.pdf.
Karshenas, M., & Moghadam, V. M. (2006). Social policy in the Middle East: Introduction and overview. In M. Karshenas & V. M. Moghadam (Eds.), *Social policy in the Middle East: Economic, political, and gender dynamics* (pp. 1–30). Basingstoke: Palgrave-Macmillan/United Nations Research Institute for Social Development.
Karshenas, M., & Moghadam, V. M. (2009). Bringing social policy back in: A look at the Middle East and North Africa. *International Journal of Social Welfare, 18*(1), 52–61.
Kwon, H. J. (2005). *The developmental welfare state and policy reforms in East Asia.* Basingstoke: Palgrave-Macmillan.
Lammy, D., & Tyler, B. C. (2014). *Wellbeing in four policy areas: Report by the all-party parliamentary group on wellbeing economics.* Retrieved from New economics foundations. http://b.3cdn.net/nefoundation/ccdf9782b6d8700f7c_lcm6i2ed7.pdf.
Massam, B. H. (2002). Quality of life: Public planning and private living. *Progress in Planning, 58,* 141–227. http://www.tlu.ee/~arro/Happy%20Space%20EKA%202014/quality%20of%20life.pdf.
McGillivray, M., & Clarke, M. (2007). Human well-being: Concepts and measures. In M. McGillivray & M. Clarke (Eds.), *Understanding human well-being* (pp. 3–16). Tokyo: United Nations University Press.
Michalos, A. C. (2004). Social indicators research and health-related quality of life research. *Social Indicators Research, 65*(1), 27–72. https://doi.org/10.1023/A:1025592219390.
Michalos, A. C. (2014). *Encyclopedia of well-being and quality of life research.* Dordrecht: Springer.
Moghadam, V. M., & Karshenas, M. (2006). *Social policy in the middle east: Economic, political, and gender dynamics.* Basingstoke: Palgrave-Macmillan/United Nations Research Institute for Social Development.
Oishi, S. (2010). Cultural and well-being: Conceptual and methodological issues. In E. Diener, et al. (Eds.), *International differences in well-being* (pp. 34–69). Oxford: Oxford University Press.
Peter, F., & Machin, D. (2015). *Quality of life.* Hoboken: Wiley.
Roy, A. (2010). *Poverty capital: Micro-finance and the making of development.* New York: Routledge.
Silva, J., Levin, V., Morgand, M. (2012). *Inclusion and resilience: The way forward for social safety nets in the Middle East and North Africa.* Washington: World Bank. Retrieved from http://citeseerx.ist.psu.edu/viewdoc/download?doi=10.1.1.372.2300&rep=rep1&type=pdf.
Sirgy, M. J. (1998). Materialism and quality of life. *Social Indicators Research, 43,* 227–260.
Sirgy, M. J. (2011). Theoretical perspectives guiding QOL indicator projects. *Social Indicators Research, 103,* 1–22.

Sirgy, M. J., Estes, R. J., & Selian, A. N. (2017). How we measure well-being: The data behind the history of well-being. In R. J. Estes & M. J. Sirgy (Eds.), *The pursuit of human well-being: The untold global history* (pp. 135–160). Dordrecht: Springer.

Theofilou, P. (2013). Quality of life: Definition and measurement. *Europe's Journal of Psychology, 9*(1), 150–162.

Tiliouine, H., & Estes, R. J. (2016). Social development in North African countries: Achievements and current challenges. In H. Tiliouine & R. J. Estes (Eds.), *The state of social progress of Islamic societies: Social, economic, political, and ideological challenges* (pp. 109–136). Dordrecht: Springer.

Tiliouine, H., & Meziane, M. (2017). The history of well-being in the Middle East and North Africa (MENA). In R. J. Estes & M. J. Sirgy (Eds.), *The Pursuit of Human Well-Being: The untold global history* (pp. 523–563). Dordrecht: Springer.

United Nations Development Programme. (2016). *Human development index.* Retrieved from http://hdr.undp.org/en/indicators/137506.

Chapter 2
Methodology

Abstract The thrust of this chapter is to designate a holistic construct using interdisciplinary and multidisciplinary approaches. In addition to scholarly literature, the study uses information collected from the world's largest data collection agencies to analyze a variety of objective and subjective indicators of well-being in the MENA region.

Keywords Methodology · Well-being indicators · Human development index

2.1 Introduction

The analysis used in this monograph is based on the social development research paradigms that place people at the center of development (Estes 1993; Lammy and Tyler 2014; Tiliouine and Estes 2016). "Sustainable development practice consists of development-focused interventions that seek to promote and enhance the social, political, and economic well-being of people" (Estes 1993: 12). It is to be noted that individuals from different cultures both view well-being and make life satisfaction judgments differently (Oishi 2010). However, the study concentrates on three constituents of the populations focused on in this book. First is the Middle East and North Africa (MENA) region itself. Second are the six countries within the MENA region selected for further analysis. Third is the global or international context within which both the MENA region as a whole and each of the selected countries are comparatively related. There is a need for the integration of local, national, regional, and global approaches.

What distinguishes this book is its strategy of addressing well-being and policy issues from multiple perspectives. Likewise, one of the distinctive features of this approach to quality of life and well-being is its interdisciplinary and multidisciplinary approaches, including social policy, development studies, public health, psychology, anthropology, history, art history, ecology, cultural geography, political science, and sociology, to mention a few (el-Aswad 2006). The simple reason for this tactic is that the study of well-being involves multiple objective and subjective measures

el-S. el-Aswad, *The Quality of Life and Policy Issues among the Middle East and North African Countries*, Human Well-Being Research and Policy Making,
https://doi.org/10.1007/978-3-030-00326-5_2

or indicators of well-being as well as multifaceted and intertwined dimensions of economic, health, educational, social, cultural, political, and personal happiness and satisfaction factors, among other dimensions.

In addition to scholarly work, the study uses information and global measures collected from the world's largest data collection and reporting agencies such as the *Human Development Index* (HDI), the *United Nations Department of Economic and Social Affairs*, the *Social Progress Index*, the UNESCO Institute for Statistics, the Freedom House, the Institute for Economics and Peace, particularly the *Global Peace Index*, the Vision of Humanity, the *Gallup Poll* (Gallup Organization), the *Global Competitiveness Index* (of the World Economic Forum), the Pew Research Center, the *Global Militarization Index*, the *World Values Survey*, and the *Global Firepower Index*. Literature on the scholarship of well-being has confirmed that composite indicators, such as the HDI, among other international indices, have been designed to challenge the hegemony of one factor or indicator such as income as the sole representative measure of human well-being (el-Aswad 2017; Huppert and Cooper 2014; McGillivray and Clarke 2007; Peter and Machin 2015; Silva et al. 2012; Sirgy 2011; Sirgy et al. 2017).

2.2 Framework

Human development needs comprise a hierarchy of basic and growth needs. Health, safety, and economic needs are essential for human survival. Social, esteem, actualization, knowledge, and aesthetics, related to human flourishing, are growth needs (Sirgy et al. 2017). The study applies the HDI, which is a composite index measuring average achievement in three basic dimensions of human development: health (life expectancy at birth), knowledge (education, including expected years of schooling and mean years of schooling), and economy (based on gross national income per capita in US dollars) (Table 2.1). The HDI "was created to emphasize that people and their capabilities should be the ultimate criteria for assessing the development of a country, not economic growth alone" (United Nations Development Programme 2016: 6).

The *United Nation Development Programme* explains the reasons behind the minimum and maximum values for each indicator. For "life expectancy," for example, the minimum of 20 years is based on the historical evidence that no country in the 20th century had a life expectancy of less than 20 years. For education, the justification for the minimum of 0 years is based on the fact that societies can subsist without formal education. The maximum of 18 years for expected years of schooling is equivalent to achieving a master's degree in most countries, whereas the maximum of 15 years for mean years of schooling is the projected maximum of this specific indicator for 2025. For gross national income per capita, the low minimum value of $100 is justified by the considerable amount of unmeasured subsistence and nonmarket production in economies close to the minimum, not attained in the official data. The maximum of $75,000 per capita is justified based on scholarly inquiries that indicate there is no gain in human development from income per capita exceeding $75,000. Currently, only two MENA countries (Kuwait and Qatar) exceed the $75,000 income per capita ceiling (Table 2.2).

Table 2.1 Indicators of well-being: Minimum and Maximum (Data from United Nation Development Index 2016)

Dimension	Indicator	Minimum	Maximum
Health	Life expectancy (years)	20	85
Education	Expected years of schooling (years)	0	18
	Mean years of schooling (years)	0	15
Standard of living	Gross national income per capita (PPP $)	100	75,000

PPP purchasing power parity

Table 2.2 Human development index, countries of the Middle East and North Africa, 2015 (Data from United Nations Development Programme 2016)

Rank	Country	Human Development Index	Life expectancy at birth	Expected years of schooling	Mean years of schooling	GDP per capita $	Population, total (millions)
	Very High Human Development						
19	Israel	0.899	82.6	16	12.8	31,215	8.1
33	Qatar	0.856	78.3	13.4	9.8	129,916	2.2
38	Saudi Arabia	0.847	74.4	16.1	9.6	51,320	31.5
42	UAE	0.84	77.1	13.3	9.5	66,203	9.2
47	Bahrain	0.824	76.7	14.5	9.4	37,236	1.4
51	Kuwait	0.8	74.5	13.3	7.3	76,075	3.9
	High Human Development						
52	Oman	0.796	77	15.7	12	34,402	4.5
69	Iran	0.774	75.6	14.8	8.8	16,395	79.1
71	Turkey	0.767	75.5	14.6	7.9	18,705	78.7
76	Lebanon	0.763	79.5	13.3	8.6	13,312	5.9
83	Algeria	0.745	75	14.4	7.8	13,533	39.7
86	Jordan	0.741	74.2	13.1	10.1	10,111	7.6
97	Tunisia	0.725	75	14.6	7.1	10,249	11.3
102	Libya	0.716	71.8	13.4	7.3	14,303	6.3
	Medium Human Development						
111	Egypt	0.691	71.3	13.1	7.1	10,250	91.5
114	Palestine	0.684	73.1	12.8	8.9	5,581	4.7
121	Iraq	0.649	69.6	10.1	6.6	11,608	36.4
123	Morocco	0.647	74.3	12.1	5	7,195	34.4
	Low Human Development						
149	Syria	0.536	69.7	9	5.1	2,441	18.5
165	Sudan	0.49	63.7	7.2	3.5	3,846	40.2
168	Yemen	0.482	64.1	9	3	2,300	26.8
	Total					**566,010**	**535.6**

GDP gross domestic product; *UAE* United Arab Emirates

It is worth nothing that the first *Report of the United Nation Human Development Index,* published in 1990, defined human development as "a process of enlarging people's choices. The most critical ones are to lead a long and healthy life, to be educated and to enjoy a decent standard of living. Additional choices include political freedom, guaranteed human rights and self-respect" (United Nations Development Programme 1990: 10). Based on this definition and where information is available and appropriate to cite, the study goes beyond the HDI framework. A variety of indicators are used to demonstrate the most crucial aspects of quality of life in the MENA region. Indicators that relate to, for instance, health, education, finance, employment, work, sports, and communication, are used in the evaluation of well-being outcomes. Indicators of quality of life deal with both objective and subjective states of well-being at both the individual and the collective levels. Objective outcome indicators refer to objective information or data collected by government and nongovernmental agencies. Indicators of subjective well-being outcomes refer to and measure states of subjective well-being such as happiness and satisfaction, which may have a strong or a weak relationship to the objective indicators of people's well-being. The main objectives of both kinds of objective and subjective indicators are to grasp the state of well-being of individuals in the context of their societies or communities. In brief, a number of indicators and measures of the objective and subjective domains of well-being are typically incorporated in the research of well-being (Cooper 2014; Galloway 2006; Helliwell et al. 2017; Huppert and Michalos 2004; Massam 2002; Sirgy et al. 2017; Theofilou 2013).

References

el-Aswad, el-S. (2006). Applied anthropology in Egypt: Practicing anthropology within local and global contexts. *National Association for the Practice of Anthropology (NAPA) Bulletin* (25), 35–51. https://doi.org/10.1525/napa.2006.25.1.035.

el-Aswad, el-S. (2017). *Well-being in the Arab world: An anthropological perspective.* Paper presented at the International Conference on Social and Related Sciences, 4–8 October. Side-Antalya, Turkey.

Estes, R. J. (1993). Toward sustainable development: From theory to praxis. *Social Development Issues, 15*(3), 1–29.

Galloway, S. (2006). Quality of life and well-being: Measuring the benefits of culture and sport: Literature review. *Scottish Executive Social Research, 12,* 3–93.

Helliwell, J. et al. (2017). *World happiness report 2017: The social foundation of world happiness* (United Nations). Retrieved from http://worldhappiness.report/wp-content/uploads/sites/2/2017/03/HR17-Ch2.pdf.

Huppert, F. A., & Cooper, C. L. (2014). *Interventions and policies to enhance wellbeing: A complete reference guide* (Vol. VI). Chichester, West Sussex: Wiley.

Lammy, D., & Tyler, B. C. (2014). *Wellbeing in four policy areas: Report by the all-party parliamentary group on wellbeing economics.* Retrieved from New Economics Foundations. http://b.3cdn.net/nefoundation/ccdf9782b6d8700f7c_lcm6i2ed7.pdf.

Massam, B. H. (2002). Quality of life: Public planning and private living. *Progress in Planning, 58,* 141–227. http://www.tlu.ee/~arro/Happy%20Space%20EKA%202014/quality%20of%20life.pdf.

McGillivray, M., & Clarke, M. (2007). Human well-being: Concepts and measures. In M. McGillivray & M. Clarke (Eds.), *Understanding human well-being* (pp. 3–16). Tokyo, New York, Paris: United Nations University Press.

Michalos, A. C. (2004). Social indicators research and health-related quality of life research. *Social Indicators Research, 65*(1), 27–72. https://doi.org/10.1023/A:1025592219390.

Oishi, S. (2010). Culture and well-being: Conceptual and methodological issues. In E. Diener et al. (Eds.), *International differences in well-being* (pp. 34–69). Oxford: Oxford University Press.

Peter, F., & Machin, D. (2015). *Quality of life*. Hoboken, NJ: Wiley.

Silva, J., Levin, V., & Morgand, M. (2012). *The way forward for social safety nets in the Middle East and North Africa.* Washington, DC: World Bank. http://citeseerx.ist.psu.edu/viewdoc/download?doi=10.1.1.372.2300&rep=rep1&type=pdf.

Sirgy, M. J. (2011). Theoretical perspectives guiding QOL indicator projects. *Social Indicators Research, 103,* 1–22.

Sirgy, M. J., Estes, R. J., & Selian, A. N. (2017). How we measure well-being: The data behind the history of well-being. In R. J. Estes & M. J. Sirgy (Eds.), *The pursuit of human well-being: The untold global history* (pp. 135–160). Dordrecht, NL: Springer.

Theofilou, P. (2013). Quality of life: Definition and measurement. *Europe's Journal of Psychology, 9*(1), 150–162.

Tiliouine, H., & Estes, R. J. (2016). Social development in North African countries: Achievements and current challenges. In H. Tiliouine & R. J. Estes (Eds.), *The state of social progress of Islamic societies: Social, economic, political, and ideological challenges* (pp. 109–136). Dordrecht, NL: Springer.

United Nation Development Programme. (1990). *Human development report.* Retrieved from http://hdr.undp.org/sites/default/files/reports/219/hdr_1990_en_complete_nostats.pdf.

United Nation Development Programme. (2016). *Human development index.* http://hdr.undp.org/en/content/human-development-index-hdi and http://hdr.undp.org/en/indicators/137506.

Chapter 3
Historical Background

Abstract This chapter discusses in broad terms the successes, challenges, quality of life, and overall human development experienced by the Middle East and North African (MENA) region from comparatively ancient to modern times. The chapter provides a rationale for identifying 21 countries as comprising the MENA region as well as for focusing on six selected countries, mainly Egypt, Iran, Israel, Tunisia, Turkey, and the United Arab Emirates. Core features of the MENA region in terms of geography, demography, economy, culture, and religion are provided. Within this historical context, the chapter addresses external and internal factors along with religious and ideological orientations impacting the quality of life in the MENA region.

Keywords MENA region · History of quality of life · Indicators of well-being Human development

3.1 Introduction

Studies addressing quality of life and well-being have increasingly grown and expanded over recent years (Daniel and Tiberius 2015; Estes and Sirgy 2018; Hamann and Rosen 2011; Kwon 2005; Lammy and Tyler 2014; Michalos 2014). Searching for acceptable measures and indicators of well-being to examine people's quality of life has become the focus of both academic researchers and policy makers in virtually all regions and countries of the world (Dawoody 2015; Hersch 2016; O'Donnell et al. 2014; Svara 2015; Wren-Lewis 2013).

This chapter examines quality of life and well-being in the different cultural contexts of the countries of the Middle East and North Africa (Silva et al. 2012), including the Gulf States (MENA) to assess shared notions of the good life and how best to achieve it. The study tackles in broad terms the well-being, successes, and challenges experienced by the MENA region from 2000 to 2015. In some selective cases, and where information is available and appropriate to cite, this study also

el-S. el-Aswad, *The Quality of Life and Policy Issues among the Middle East and North African Countries*, Human Well-Being Research and Policy Making,
https://doi.org/10.1007/978-3-030-00326-5_3

briefly discusses well-being in terms of economy, health, and education in the ancient, medieval, and modern history of the MENA region.

The concepts of "quality of life" and "well-being" are not the same for all people, past or present, or for those living under different social conditions. Public policy to address well-being becomes necessary when people and nations as a whole need help improving their quality of life. Public policy here indicates the process or means through which a government acts to improve people's quality of life or deals with the needs of its citizens via plans and actions defined by the law or its constitution. Public policy affects a portion of the public (Hersch 2016; Jawad 2015; Lammy and Tyler 2014; O'Donnell et al. 2014; Svara 2015; Wren-Lewis 2013). Private policy can be viewed as a plan or policy, not free of regulation, that is created and implemented by non-governmental organizations and voluntary or non-profit agencies to promote societal and individual well-being (Estes and Zhou 2015; Hersch 2016; Thompson 1983).

One of the core objectives of well-being studies is to provide reliable information to assist policy makers to realize critical aspects of human development that otherwise would be less visible. To arrive at well-informed decisions on how best to promote quality of life and well-being, policy makers need to know how different policies affect well-being. Quality of life is a multidimensional concept that refers to the physical, mental, and social wellness that goes beyond the traditional concept of economic well-being (Estes and Sirgy 2017; Sirgy et al. 2017).

3.2 The Middle East and North Africa Region

"Regions are defined as countries that are close to one another geographically and, in most cases, share a common set of social and economic characteristics" (Sirgy et al. 2017: 146). Historically, the term *Middle East* goes back to the early 20th century, indicating a "Western" geographic construct stemming from the security studies of Admiral Alfred Thayer Mahan and others, which were used extensively in the United States after the Second World War (Keddie 1973). Several scholars provide broader definitions of the Middle East in geographical terms including through the use of maps and figures (Bonine et al. 2011). However, definitions contingent on current nation-states are common and recognizable where these countries are members of the United Nations.

The United Nations Department of Economic and Social Affairs does not designate MENA countries as comprising a unified region. However, although there is no universally agreed upon definition of the MENA region and its geographic boundary because it is large and diverse, this study views the region as expanding from Morocco in the west to Iran in the east, and from Turkey in the north to Sudan in the south. Because the MENA region is large and diverse, this research adopts certain criteria related particularly to culture, economy, and population. For example, although income distribution in Arabian Gulf countries is relatively similar, populations and perceptions among their residents and citizens are significantly different as is the case with Saudi Arabia and Qatar. Therefore, this study pursues both broad and focused approaches. Broadly, this inquiry addresses 21 MENA countries, which alphabetically include Algeria, Bahrain, Egypt, Iran, Iraq, Israel, Jordan, Kuwait, Lebanon, Libya, Morocco, Oman, Palestine, Qatar, Saudi Arabia, Sudan, Syria, Tunisia, Turkey, the United Arab Emirates, and Yemen. The focus (in the following chapters) is analytically and comparatively on six countries: Egypt, Iran, Israel, Turkey, Tunisia, and the UAE.

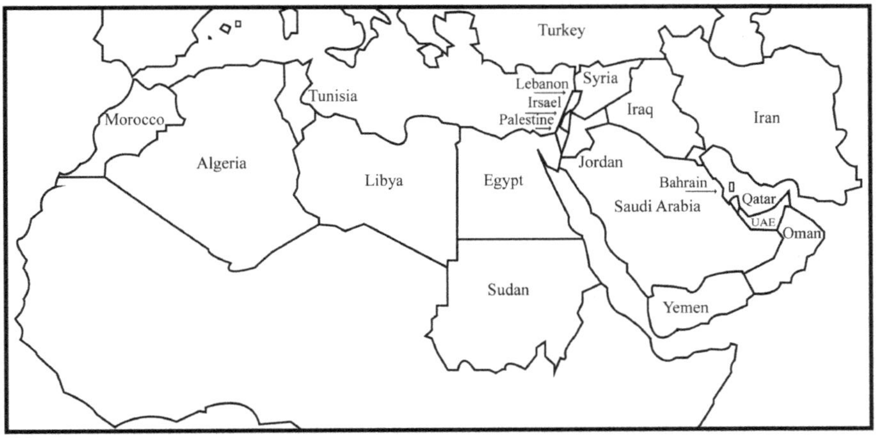

Map of the Middle East and North African region, drawn by Amir El-Aswad

These six countries represent the MENA region in multiple and significant domains including, for example, economy, culture, language, demography, geographic location, and political system. In terms of geographical size and population, they include three large countries (Egypt, Iran, and Turkey) comprising more than 50% of the total population of the MENA region and three small countries (Israel, Tunisia, and the UAE). In terms of geographic location, two countries (Egypt and Tunisia) are located in North Africa, three countries (Israel, Iran, and Turkey) are located in Asia, and one country (the UAE) is located in the Arabian Gulf region. Regarding language, the selected countries represent the main formal languages of Arabic, Hebrew, Persian, and Turkish. In terms of economy or gross domestic product (GDP) per capita, these countries include some of the world's widest income disparities, as in the case of Egypt (medium income) and the UAE (very high income), for example. They also represent the MENA region in terms of the United Nations Human Development Index (HDI), which classifies countries based on the categories of very high human development (Israel and the UAE), high human development (Iran, Tunisia, and Turkey), medium human development (Egypt), and low human development. All of these key features make the selected countries suitable to this study.

The central location of the MENA region between Europe, Africa, and Asia implies that MENA countries are still a focus of attention. In addition to Iran and

Turkey, the MENA region is known to include three subregions: The Gulf Cooperation Council (GCC), the Levant, and North Africa. The MENA region enjoys strategic locations including geographic positions that connect the continents of Africa, Asia, and Europe. Additionally, some nations such as Egypt and Turkey are considered transcontinental countries. Whereas Egypt stretches from Africa into Asia, Turkey stretches from Asia into Europe. The official languages in the MENA region include Arabic, Hebrew, Persian (Farsi), and Turkish. Other languages of ethnic groups include, for instance, Berber or Amazigh, Chaldean, and Kurdish, among others (Suleiman 2013).

The world's major oil reserves are located in the MENA region (World Energy Council 2016). Eight out of the fourteen oil-exporting Organization of the Petroleum Exporting Countries are located in the MENA region (Algeria, Iran, Iraq, Kuwait, Libya, Qatar, Saudi Arabia, and the UAE). Four out of the five founders of Organization of the Petroleum Exporting Countries, founded in Baghdad in 1960, were MENA countries (Iran, Iraq, Kuwait, and Saudi Arabia).

The MENA region encompasses different political systems. For example, the states of the Arabian Gulf, Jordan, and Morocco are monarchies; the rest of the MENA counties are republics and use electoral systems. In the GCC, the formation of civil society and the institutional formation of the modern state have not been fully materialized as government dominates political life. Political loyalty is key for the government's handouts (*makrama*). People rely more heavily on the ruling nobility or government than on themselves (Lee 2010).

3.3 Population

Population is an essential consideration for well-being studies. When the size of a country's population increases, greater demands are placed on economic resources and social services to accommodate population growth. The annual growth rate reached 2.2%, twice the global population growth rate of 1%. The MENA region is characterized by a young population representing around 30% of the total population (Organization for Economic Co-operation and Development 2016). Although some countries such as Iran, Turkey, Lebanon, and Tunisia, following population policies, managed to lower their fertility rates to the replacement level of 2.1 per woman in 2015, fertility issues need to be managed in other countries such Israel, Egypt, Yemen, Sudan, and Iraq, whose fertility rates in 2015 were 3.1, 3.4, 4.4, 4.5, and 4.6 children per woman, respectively. According to the HDI, the total population of the 21 MENA countries (selected for this study) was estimated in 2015 to be around 536 million people, comprising about 7.5% of the total world population (United Nations Development Programme 2016a) (Table 2.2).

MENA countries vary in population size, natural resources, economies, geographic size, and standards of living. The population growth in the region is among the highest in the world. As a result of the rapid population growth, age structure in the MENA region is very different from that in Western Europe (Maddison 2007).

Most of the MENA countries, particularly Egypt, Iran, and Turkey, are rapidly growing. For example, the population of Egypt in 2000 was 67.9 million and increased to 91.5 million in 2015. Similarly, Iran's population was 67.2 million in 2000 and increased to 79.1 million in 2015. The population of Turkey was 66.7 million in 2001, reaching 78.7 million in 2015. Together (Egypt, Iran, and Turkey) with Algeria and the Sudan, these five most populated countries comprise about 65% of the region's population (Tables 2.2 and 3.1). In addition, the MENA region is characterized by the fastest-growing urban populations in the world, with approximately 70% of inhabitants living in cities. The region's two mega cities (defined as more than 10 million people) are Cairo, with 18 million, and Istanbul, with 14 million (Keulertz et al. 2016).

Even a small country such as the UAE has experienced a rapid growth in population, reaching 9.2 million in 2015 compared to 2.9 million in 2000. Although the increase of the population in Egypt is not impacted by migration, Israel and the UAE show a different pattern. For example, migrants and expatriates comprise more than 90% of the UAE population. To increase the local population of the Emirati nationals, the UAE government founded what is known as the Marriage Fund, established by Federal Law No. 47 of 1992, allowing UAE national male grooms of at least 21 years of age to apply for a 70,000.00 United Arab Emirates Dirhams ($19,058) marriage grant so as to marry an Emirati female of at least 18 years of age. In addition, the UAE government continues to financially persuade Emirati families to have more children by offering 600 United Arab Emirates Dirhams ($164.00) a month to a male citizen to whom a child is born (el-Aswad 2012). According to Federal Law No. 2 of 2001, monthly assistance is provided to the following categories of UAE nationals residing within the UAE: widows, divorcees, disabled or those with special needs, elderly, orphans, children from unknown parents, medically unfit persons, married students, families of prisoners, financially unfit persons, abandoned women, and UAE national women married to expatriate men who cannot earn a living for reasons beyond their control (United Arab Emirates Government 2018).

Mass immigration plays a crucial role in the state building of Israel where the vast scope of the immigration relative to the size of the host population is "unheard of in any immigrant country" (Shapira 2012: 183). Because of the mass immigration, the number of Jews living in Israel more than doubled between 1948 and 1951 (Lee 2010: 84). In 2000, Israel's population was 6 million, but it increased to 8.1 million in 2015 (Tables 2.2 and 3.1).

3.4 Overall Human Development

All MENA countries "started with a very low social development base in the post-Second World War period ... Average under five-infant mortality in the region was over 300 per 1000 in 1960, the average of life expectancy in the late 1960s was about 50, and adult illiteracy was at staggering 65 percent, even as late as 1970" (Karshenas and Moghadam 2009: 64). By 1990s, most MENA countries had shown

Table 3.1 Human Development Index of the countries of the Middle East and North Africa, 2000 (Data from the Human Development Report [United Nations Development Programme 2002])

Rank	Country	Human Development Index	Life expectancy at birth	Adult literacy rate (% age 15 and above)	Combined primary, secondary, and tertiary gross enrolment ratio	Education Index	GDP per capita (US$)	Population, total (millions)
	High Human Development							
22	Israel	0.896	78.7	94.6	83	0.91	20,131	6
39	Bahrain	0.831	73.7	87.6	80	0.85	15,084	0.3
45	Kuwait	0.813	76.2	82	59	0.74	15,799	1.9
46	UAE	0.812	75	76.3	68	0.74	33,071	2.9
51	Qatar	0.803	69.6	81.2	75	0.79	18,789	0.2
	Medium Human Development							
64	Libya	0.773	70.5	80	92	0.84	7570	5.3
71	Saudi Arabia	0.759	71.6	76.3	70	0.83	11,360	20.3
75	Lebanon	0.755	73.1	86	78	0.83	4308	3.5
78	Oman	0.751	71	71.7	58	0.67	13,356	2.5
85	Turkey	0.742	69.8	85.1	62	0.77	12,815	66.7
97	Tunisia	0.722	73.2	71	74	0.73	7386	9.5
98	Iran	0.717	68.9	76.3	73	0.77	11,894	67.2
99	Jordan	0.741	70.3	89.7	55	0.78	3966	4.9
106	Algeria	0.697	69.6	66.7	72	0.74	5308	30.3
108	Syria	0.688	71.2	74.4	63	0.71	3556	16.2
115	Egypt	0.642	67.3	55.3	76	0.62	7629	67.9
123	Morocco	0.602	67.6	48.9	52	0.5	3546	29.9
	Low Human Development							
139	Sudan	0.499	56	57.8	34	0.5	1797	31.1
144	Yemen	0.479	60.6	46.3	51	0.48	893	18.3

GDP Gross domestic product

improvement in the domains of health care as presented in health indicators including life expectancy and infant mortality" (Karshenas and Moghadam 2009: 65).

MENA countries have achieved significant progress in the overall Human Development Indices of 2000 and 2015 in the domains of health, education, and economy. The HDI of 2000 classified 173 countries (including the MENA region) into 3 categories: 1 = high human development (with an HDI of 80 or above); 2 = medium human development (50–79); and 3 = low human development (less than 50).

In HDI 2000, five MENA countries (Bahrain, Israel, Kuwait, Qatar, and the UAE) were included in the 53 countries achieving a high rank (above a score of 80). Israel ranked 1 among MENA countries and 22 worldwide; Bahrain ranked 2 among MENA countries and 39 worldwide; Kuwait ranked 3 among MENA countries and 45 worldwide; the UAE ranked 4 among MENA countries and 46 globally; and Qatar ranked 5 among MENA countries and 51 worldwide. Twelve MENA countries out of 134 countries achieved the rank of medium human development. These countries include Algeria, Egypt, Iran, Jordan, Lebanon, Libya, Morocco, Oman, Saudi Arabia, Syria, Tunisia, and Turkey. Two countries, the Sudan and Yemen, were rated low in human development (ranked, respectively, 139 and 144 worldwide). Data of two countries, Iraq and Palestine, are not provided in the HDI (Table 3.1).

In the HDI of 2015, countries were classified into 4 categories: 1 = very high human development (with an HDI score of 80 or above); 2 = high human development (HDI score of 70–79); 3 = medium human development (HDI score of 55–69); and 4 = low human development (HDI score less than 55). According to the 2015 HDI (United Nations Development Programme 2016b), six MENA countries (Bahrain, Israel, Kuwait, Qatar, Saudi Arabia, and the UAE) were included in the 51 countries ranked very high in human development. Israel ranked first among the MENA countries and 19 worldwide. Qatar, the richest country with $129,916 per capita, ranked 2 among the MENA countries and 33 worldwide. Saudi Arabia, moving from a medium rank in 2000, ranked 3 among the MENA countries and 38 globally. The UAE rated 4 among MENA countries and 41 worldwide; Bahrain ranked 5 among MENA countries and 47 globally, whereas Kuwait rated 6 among MENA countries and 51 worldwide (Table 2.2).

Eight MENA countries were among the 53 countries that ranked high. These countries were Algeria, Iran, Jordan, Lebanon, Libya, Oman, Tunisia, and Turkey. Four MENA countries (Egypt, Palestine, Iraq, and Morocco) were among the 41 countries that ranked medium. And, three MENA countries (Syria, Sudan, and Yemen) were among the 53 countries who ranked low (Table 2.2).

Individual or household income is positively related to well-being and life satisfaction within and between countries (Deaton 2008; Diener et al. 1993, p. 201; Huppert and Cooper 2014). Economically, the total GDP per capita of the MENA region (21 countries being studied) was $566,010 in 2015 and the average GDP per capita of the region was $15,572, which was slightly lower than the world's GDP per capita of $16,000 (Central Intelligence Agency 2016). Between the years 2000 and 2015, incomes generally increased in the MENA countries, especially those not the recipient of current military intervention. For instance, whereas the GDP per capita of Qatar increased seven times from $18,789 in 2000 to $129,916 in 2015 (ranked first

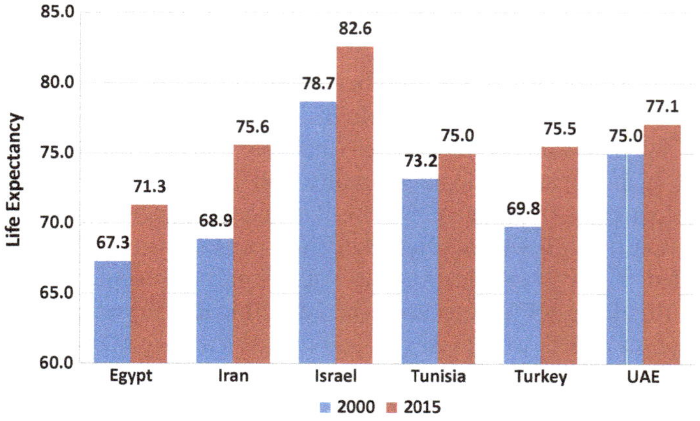

Fig. 3.1 Life expectancy in selected Middle Eastern and North African countries, 2000–2015 UAE = United Arab Emirates (Data from United Nations Development Programme 2002, 2016b)

both regionally and globally), the GDP per capita of Kuwait increased five times from $15,799 in 2000 to $76,075 in 2015. Israel's GDP per capita also increased; it was $20,131 in 2000 and reached $31,215 in 2015. Although states such as Turkey, whose GDP per capita tripled from $6974 in 2001 to $18,705 in 2015, and Egypt, whose GDP per capita improved from $6090 in 2001 to $10,064 in 2015, other MENA countries, such as Syria and Yemen, failed to advance in income (Tables 2.2 and 3.1). Such cases indicate that inequalities in income influence inequalities in other dimensions of well-being and vice versa (United Nations Development Programme 2016b).

Good health or healthy related behavior is strongly associated with good quality of life and well-being (Ellison and Smith 1991; Huppert and Cooper 2014; Peter and Machin 2015). Concerning health issues in the MENA region, indicators show that there has been progress in health care among most of the MENA countries where the longevity or "life expectancy at birth" has improved (World Health Organization 2017). For instance, in Israel, life expectancy at birth was 78.7 years in 2000, and it reached 82.6 years in 2015. Although the average age of the Lebanese in 2000 was 71.6 years, it increased to 79.5 years in 2015. Among the Qatari, the average age improved from 69.6 years in 2000 to 78.3 years in 2015. The average age in Iran was 68.9 years in 2000 but increased to 75.6 years in 2015 (Tables 2.2 and 3.1). There is also significant improvement in the selected MENA countries (between 2000 and 2015) as shown in Fig. 3.1. However, some countries that have suffered from political conflict and civil war such as Syria and Libya, have experienced a grave regression in terms of longevity.

Quality of education is important in making learning enjoyable and promoting social well-being (Estes 2017; Huppert and Cooper 2014). The progress of education among MENA countries has varied. According to the Human Development Indices of 2000 and 2015, education has improved in several MENA countries. For example, the indicator of "expected years of schooling" increased in Israel from 14.7 years in 2000 to 16 years in 2015. It reached 16.1 years in Saudi Arabia in 2015. The "expected years of schooling" slightly developed in Palestine from 11.4 years in 2000 to 13.1 years in 2015, whereas in Morocco it increased from 9.2 years in 2000 to 12.1 years in 2015. In 2015, the indicator of "mean years of schooling" was 12.8 in Israel, 12.0 in Oman, and 10.1 in Jordan (Tables 2.2 and 3.1). Despite these successes, the MENA countries failed to establish robust foundations for democratic systems of governance and failed to settle the Arab-Israeli conflict and deal with other critical ethnic and religious issues (Tiliouine and Meziane 2017). It should be noted that international data show a positive relationship between democratic institutions and life satisfaction (Huppert and Cooper 2014).

3.5 Brief History

The history of the MENA region, the cradle of ancient civilizations, is long, rich, and multilayered. It is impossible to portray a single picture of the well-being in MENA countries, given the vast diversity of historical, political, and economic features they have experienced as well as the various cultural characteristics they possess.

3.5.1 The Quality of Life in the Ancient MENA Region

Agricultural societies, which preceded literate urban civilizations, flourished in Egypt, Mesopotamia (Iraq), Persia, (Iran), Turkey, and the countries of the Levant. With their early domestication of plants and animals, these agricultural societies were the source of the European Neolithic period (Derricourt 2015). Ancient MENA civilizations recognized that ideological, religious, political, and hierarchical systems governing civil service classes were beneficial in securing effective means for promoting the well-being of MENA populations.

In ancient Egypt, the well-being of the society was contingent on the pursuit of ma'at, an ethical principle of justice, truth, or "what is right" that, according to the Pyramid Texts of Unas, goes back to 2375 Before the Common Era (BCE). Egyptian people were expected to pursue ma'at throughout their daily lives to achieve and maintain their well-being at levels of the person, the family, the nation, and the deity. The highest and divine authority such as the king was entitled to create and maintain ma'at to help people to behave or do and say "what is right" (Quirke 2015). According to archaic Egyptian cosmology, there are "two intermingled and inseparable themes associated with two dominant and overarching sovereigns. One theme deals with natural cosmology or cosmogony as associated with the sun god Ra, while the other concerns social cosmology that treats social and political relationships as well as the dilemma of life and death closely connected to the slain god Osiris. These two interconnected forms of natural and social cosmologies indicate a significant development of ancient Egyptians' thought and worldviews" (el-Aswad 1997, p. 70). The Egyptians believed their king to be the embodiment of ma'at, which resulted in the well-being of everyone (Chadwick 2005). Akhenaten, who died in 1335 BCE, qualified his name with the phrase "Living in ma'at" (Chadwick 2005). In the thirteenth century BCE, the pharaohs of the 19th Dynasty built the city of Ramses in the eastern Delta as their residence. The city was described as a place of good life, prosperity, and health (Orlin 2007). Concerning health care, Egyptians established the practice of physical examination, diagnosis, and remedies in their primary care practices. Herodotus (c. 484–425 BCE), the ancient Greek historian, described the Egyptians as the healthiest of all people, along with the Libyans (Tiliouine and Estes 2016).

Egypt was the richest part of the MENA region because of the special character of its agriculture, which yielded a large surplus of wealth for governance and monument-building in pharaonic times (Maddison 2007). In discussing the economy and population of Africa, Maddison (2007) states that, for about four millennia, Egypt was virtually the only area to practice agriculture; the rest of the continent was sparsely inhabited by hunter-gatherer populations. In the first century of the Common Era (CE), the MENA region was under Roman rule. Egypt was the most prosperous area, with a relatively large urban population (Maddison 2003). In the first millennium, the population of Egypt reached 4000, whereas the population of other countries of North Africa was about 4200 (Maddison 2007).

The concept of well-being in ancient Mesopotamian was based on ideological, religious, institutional, and economic hierarchies dealing with existential concerns or issues. The existential concerns included two parts: one was intrinsic or fundamental to the life and well-being of the individual; the other was contingent or social, concerning both the individual and society. Whereas fundamental concerns related to reproduction, birth, death, and health, contingent issues related to social vigor, success, wealth, security, and prestige (Maisels 1993). Hammurabi, the sixth king of the Old Babylonian Dynasty, who ruled Mesopotamia between 1792 and 1750 BCE, was depicted as the "King of Justice," a ruler whose duty was to keep the society in good order as well as to oversee the economic balance between the rich and the poor (Orlin 2007: 18–19).

Ancient Palestine was viewed as a "land of milk and honey" (Orlin 2007). The location of the Hebrew kingdom, between 1050 and 930 BCE, between Asia Minor and Egypt, enabled local leaders to conduct economic exchange and profit from commerce between these areas. For example, fine horses were brought from Anatolia, and excellent chariots were brought from Egypt (Orlin 2007).

3.5.2 *The Quality of Life in the Medieval Era*

Because of its strategic location connecting three continents with the major commercial networks, the MENA region was prosperous, representing the world's leading economic power from the 7th to the 12th centuries (Maddison 2007).

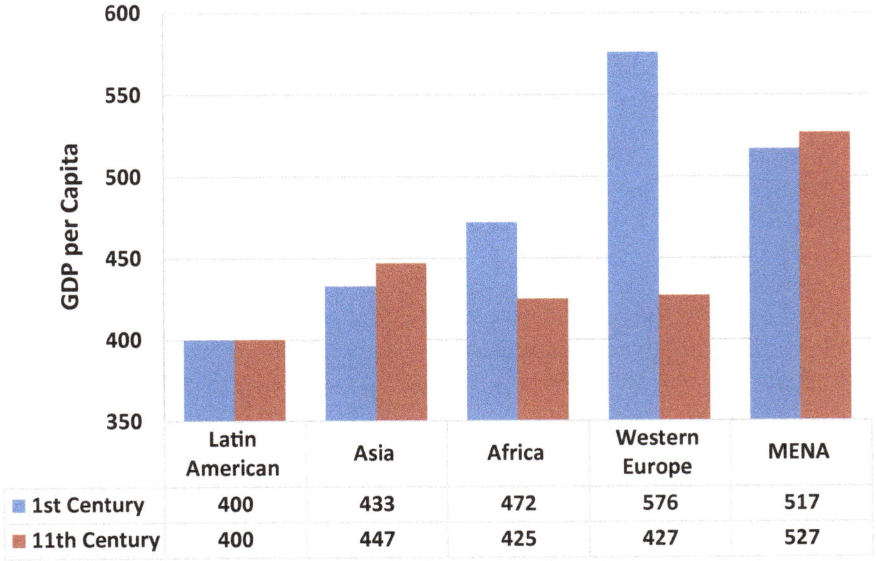

Fig. 3.2 Gross domestic product per capita in the first and the eleventh centuries (international Geary-Khamis dollars) MENA = Middle East and North America (Data from Maddison 2003, 2007)

Figure 3.2 shows that the GDP per capita in the MENA region in the 11th century was the highest of the five regions.

The Medieval era is known as the "Golden Age" of Islam during which great developments in the domains of economy, education, science, art, and the humanities were accomplished by the Abbasid Dynasty (750 CE–1258 CE) centered in Baghdad, the Fatimid Dynasty (909 CE–1171 CE) based in Cairo, and the Andalusian Dynasties (711 CE–1492 CE) based in Spain. The Golden Age of Islam coincided with the period of the European Dark Ages (500 CE–1000 CE) through to the period of the European Renaissance, between the 13th and 15th centuries (Renima et al. 2016).

In the domain of culture and education, the MENA countries contributed to the region's well-being through many significant innovations in art, mathematics, technology, literature, and architecture, bringing unprecedented affluence and prosperity to a large percentage of the MENA population. Between the 13th and the 19th centuries, the House of Wisdom (Bait Al-Hikmah), founded in Baghdad, provided a remarkable cultural arena in which Muslim, Christian, and Jewish scholars, among persons of other cultural backgrounds, made significant contributions to science, art, and philosophy (Gutas 1998). During this period, encyclopedic works of Ibn Sīnā, Ibn Rushd, Muhammed Ibn Mūsa al-Khāwrizmī, Ibn al-Haitham, Abu Rayḥān al-Bīrūnī, al-Fārābī, and al-Kindī, to mention a few, contributed to the advancement of knowledge and science (Estes and Tiliouine 2014; Fowden 2013; Gutas 1998; Renima et al. 2016).

3.5.3 The Quality of Life in Modern History

The quality of life and socioeconomic and political systems of most MENA countries have been deeply impacted by imperial and colonial forces. Before the First World War, much of the MENA region was under Ottoman, British, and French forces. For instance, in 18th and 19th centuries, the French invaded Egypt (in 1798) and occupied Algeria (in 1830) and Tunisia (in 1881) (Abun-Nasr 1987; McDougall 2011). British forces attacked Egypt in 1882 and since then "Egypt had been a de facto British colonial protectorate, a status that was confirmed in 1922" (Ballantyne and Burton 2012). The British intervention in the Arabian Gulf in 1809 led to the transformation of local sheikhdoms to Trucial States (previously named by the British as the Pirate Coast) under the British protectorate in the mid-1800s (Commins 2012; McDougall 2011). During the First World War, the Sykes-Picot Agreement was made in 1916 between the British and French Allies, mandating and colonizing Middle East countries: the British would acquire Iraq, the French would control Syria and Lebanon, and Palestine would become an international territory (Schneer 2010). But, the Balfour declaration of 1917, proclaiming the establishment of a National Jewish Home in Palestine, triggered an ongoing Israeli–Palestinian conflict (Schneer 2010) (Table 3.2). The Israel's new Nationality Law, passed in the Knesset in July 19, 2018, is viewed as a violation of principles of equality and democracy as it depicts non-Jewish citizens of Israel, especially its Arab and Druze citizens, as not part of the nation (Pappe 2018; Richman 2018).

A positive aspect in the MENA region during the 18th and 19th centuries was that "millets," or minorities, such as Armenians, Christians, Greeks, and Jews, played an important part in the economic, educational, and industrial development in countries such as Egypt, Lebanon, Syria, Turkey, Iran, Palestine, Morocco, and Algeria (Issawi 1982). Minorities had the habit of helping and promoting each other, and they participated in developing sectors of the economy, particularly foreign trade with the West, but also finance, mechanized transport, modern industry, and export-oriented agriculture. In addition, "they improved in learning both foreign languages and technical skills, which made them more employable in private and government sectors as well as in foreign enterprises" (Issawi 1982: 89) (Table 3.2).

3.6 Well-Being and Challenges Since 1950

The previous section provided a discussion of the impact of external factors, particularly colonialism, on well-being in the MENA countries. Since then, social progress in the MENA region has been challenged by both external and internal factors. In the 1950s and 1960s, most of MENA countries were concerned with issues of decolonization, national independence, and the liberation of Palestine. However, independence brought many serious challenges. Most of the MENA nation-states were new with new political elites seeking to secure legitimacy and achieve political stability. They

Table 3.2 The modern history of events affecting well-being of selected countries of the Middle East and North Africa (Central Intelligence Agency 2016)

Year	World	Egypt	Iran	Israel	Tunisia	Turkey	UAE
1798		French forces invade Egypt					
1801		British and Turkish forces repel French occupation					
1805		Muhammad Ali, an Ottoman Albanian officer, founds his dynasty					
1820							General Marine Treaty of Peace between Britain and local rulers
1831					French occupation		
1853							Trucial States based on a treaty between Britain and local sheiks
1861–65	U.S. Civil War						
1869		Suez Canal opens					

(continued)

Table 3.2 (continued)

Year	World	Egypt	Iran	Israel	Tunisia	Turkey	UAE
1876						The Ottoman ruler, Sultan Abdul Hamid II, assumes control of the empire	
1882		British forces take control of Egypt					
1892							Exclusivity Treaty between Britain and Trucial States starting the British dominance over the region
1914	Outbreak of World War I	Egypt becomes a British protectorate				The Ottoman Empire enters World War I on the side of the Central Powers	
1916	Sykes-Picot Agreement dividing and controlling MENA						

(continued)

Table 3.2 (continued)

Year	World	Egypt	Iran	Israel	Tunisia	Turkey	UAE
1917	Russian revolution			Balfour Declaration			
1918	End of World War I					Collapse of Ottoman Empire	
1922	USSR established	Egypt gains independence (end of British protectorate), although British military presence remains until 1954					
1923						Republic of Turkey is established	
1924						The Ottoman caliphate is abolished by the Turkish Grand National Assembly	
1925			Pahlavi Monarchy				
1928		Foundation of Muslim Brotherhood				Turkey becomes secular	

(continued)

Table 3.2 (continued)

Year	World	Egypt	Iran	Israel	Tunisia	Turkey	UAE
1939	Outbreak of World War II						
1945	End of World War II	Arab League, formed in Cairo on 22 March 1945 with six members (currently, 22 members)					
1947				United Nations recommends partition of Palestine into separate Jewish and Arab states			
1948				The state of Israel is proclaimed			
1948				First Arab-Israeli war			
1951			Nationalization of oil industry				
1952		Egyptian Revolution				Turkey becomes a NATO member country	The seven emirates form a Trucial Council
1956		Nationalization of the Suez Canal		Israel, Britain, and France invade Egypt	Independence		

(continued)

Table 3.2 (continued)

Year	World	Egypt	Iran	Israel	Tunisia	Turkey	UAE
1957					End of monarchy—becomes a republic		
1962							Oil is exported from Abu Dhabi
1967		Six-Day War: Israel launches a preemptive attack on Egypt, Syria, and Jordan		Israel seizes Sinai and Gaza Strip from Egypt, the Golan Heights from Syria, and the West Bank and East Jerusalem from Jordan			
1968							Britain announces it will end the protectorate in 1971
1971			Iran occupies the islands of Greater Tunb, Lesser Tunb, and Abu Musa (November)				UAE: Abu Dhabi, Dubai, Sharjah, Fujairah, Ajman, and Umm al-Quwain
1972							Ras al-Khaimah joins the UAE

(continued)

Table 3.2 (continued)

Year	World	Egypt	Iran	Israel	Tunisia	Turkey	UAE
1973		October War with Israel in which parts of Sinai are restored		The Yom Kippur War			
1979		Egypt and Israel sign a peace treaty					
1979			Islamic Revolution				
1979			The Islamic Republic of Iran is proclaimed				
1980			Start of Iran-Iraq war				
1981	Foundation of GCC						UAE is a founding member of the GCC
1982			Egypt restores the last occupied portion of Sinai	Israel invades Lebanon in order to expel Palestine Liberation Organization Massacre of Palestinians in the Sabra and Shatila camps in Beirut			

(continued)

Table 3.2 (continued)

Year	World	Egypt	Iran	Israel	Tunisia	Turkey	UAE
1985				Israel withdraws from most of Lebanon			
1987	Al-Qaeda, a global network of Islamic extremists, designated by the United Nations Security Council as a terrorist group			Intifada uprising begins in Occupied Territories	Military coup led by Zine El Abidine Ben Ali who becomes president		
1988			End of Iran-Iraq war				
1990			Iran and Iraq resume diplomatic ties				
1991	Gulf War— US led coalition to liberate Kuwait from Iraqi occupation	Egyptian forces join the coalition against Iraq's invasion of Kuwait					UAE forces join the coalition against Iraq's invasion of Kuwait
1994				Israel withdraws from most of Gaza and West Bank			

(continued)

Table 3.2 (continued)

Year	World	Egypt	Iran	Israel	Tunisia	Turkey	UAE
1994				Israel and Jordan sign a peace treaty			
1996						Pro-Islamist Welfare Party heads the government	
1998						Pro-Islamist Welfare Party banned	
2001	Sept. 11 attack destroying New York World Trade Center						
2002			Iran, Iraq, and North Korea are viewed by US as an "axis of evil"			Islamist-based Justice and Development Party (AK) wins election victory	
2003	United States attacks Iraq						
2007			International Atomic Energy Agency states Iran could develop a nuclear weapon				

(continued)

Table 3.2 (continued)

Year	World	Egypt	Iran	Israel	Tunisia	Turkey	UAE
2008	Global economic crisis			Invasion of Gaza to prevent Hamas from launching rockets			
2010			Fourth round of sanctions against Iran imposed by UN Security Council	The Gaza flotilla raid (in international waters in the Mediterranean Sea) in which Turkish pro-Palestinian activists are killed, resulting in Israel-Turkey tensions	Protests break out in December against corruption		
2011	Arab Spring in 5 MENA countries	Collapse of Mubarak regime in February			President Zine El Abidine Ben Ali goes into exile in January	Unrest in Syria caused thousands of refugees to flee to Turkey	
2012		Muslim Brotherhood regime					

(continued)

Table 3.2 (continued)

Year	World	Egypt	Iran	Israel	Tunisia	Turkey	UAE
2013	Islamic State or IS (former ISIS), a global- terrorist group aimed at creating a caliphate across Iraq, Syria, and beyond	End of Muslim Brotherhood regime/Egypt's interim government					
2014		Election of a new president					
2015			Nuclear deal with world powers (5 + 1)			Tension between Turkey-Syria borders caused by IS terrorist group	UAE joins Saudi Arabia-led coalition against Yemen (Houthis)
2016				Israel-Turkey agreement over 2010 Gaza flotilla raid and normalization of relations		Turkish President Recep Tayyip Erdogan blames US-based cleric Fethullah Gülen for an attempted coup	

GCC Gulf Cooperation Council, *IS* Islamic State, *MENA* Middle East and North Africa, *NATO* North Atlantic Treaty Organization, *UAE* United Arab Emirates, *US* United States reinforced their legitimacy by employing despotism or by creating one-party states with rulers with no term limits—keeping their position for life at the expense of people' freedom (Freedom House 2017: Maddison 2007).

3.6.1 External Factors

In the 1950s and 1960s while most MENA countries were concerned with the issues of decolonization, national independence and the liberation of Palestine, many countries were subsequently reduced to fragmented and dependent states by old and new imperialism including wars, the expansion of the global market economy, privatization, labor migration, the use of multiple media and the Internet, and global violence. "The postcolonial world is one in which we may live after colonialism but never without it" (Dirks 1992: 23). Imperial and global agents, with the strategy to divide and rule, manipulated ethnic and religious divisions that not only aggravated socioeconomic and political problems in the MENA region such as instability, poverty, unemployment, homelessness, religious sectarianism, and violence, but also lead to serious outcomes concerning indigenous cultures and identities of MENA nations (el-Aswad 2006, 2016a).

To be more specific, conflicting global and regional powers triggered broader economic, social, and political problems that aggravated the deteriorating conditions of social progress and well-being in the MENA region at large. According to the Pew Global Attitudes survey (Pew Research Center 2011), a median of 53% of Muslims surveyed, mostly from the MENA region, asserted that U.S. and Western policies were one of the main reasons why Muslim nations are lagging behind in economic prosperity and well-being.

The following are a few examples of the current negative impact of external forces on the quality of life in the MENA region. The US military invasion and occupation of Iraq in 2003 has had an ongoing negative impact on economic and political life. Although the regime in Iraq monopolized the government system before the invasion, the Shi'a and Kurds, after the invasion, dominated the political landscape at the expense of the majority Sunni (el-Aswad 2016a). Another example is that with the support of Qatari military troops, air strikes of Libya by the North Atlantic Treaty Organization in 2011 left the country divided by diverse malicious militias armed with heavy military equipment (The Guardian 2011). Yet another example is the destabilization of Syria. Conflicting forces occupy much of Syria: global forces (United States/European Union Vs. Russia), regional (Arab Gulf countries Vs. Iran) forces, and local (affiliated rebel groups pro and against the Assad regime) forces have managed to create so much devastation and destruction, making Syria a failed state. Figure 3.3 shows that life expectancy in Syria dropped from 71.5 years in 2001 to 69.7 in 2015. Similarly, the average age of Libyans decreased from 72.4 years in 2001 to 71.8 in 2015 (United Nations Development Programme 2003, 2016a).

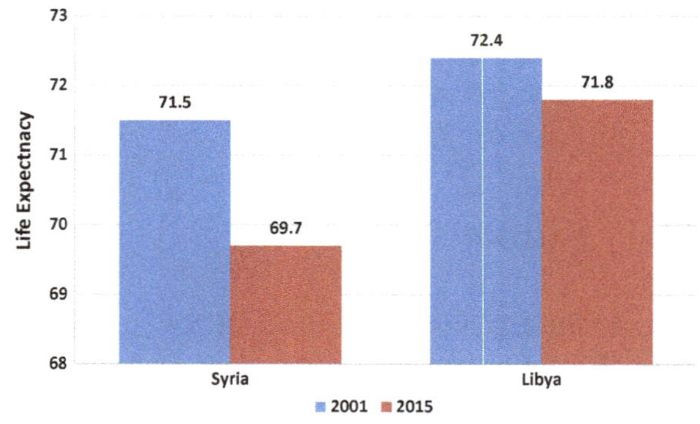

Fig. 3.3 Life expectancy at birth (Syria and Libya) (Data from Human Development Reports [United Nations Development Programme 2003, 2016a])

3.6.2 Internal Factors

Economic and political conditions in most MENA countries pose policy challenges for achieving a good quality of life. Examples include the Israeli–Palestinian or Arab–Israeli conflict, resulting in three deadly wars (1948, 1967, and 1973); the Iraq invasion of Kuwait, Turkey, and the Gulf involvement in Syria's civil war; the Saudi Arabia-Iran conflict; the Saudi-led intervention in Yemen; and the rise of the self-declared Islamic State (IS), previously ISIS or Da'ish (developed from Al-Qa'ida in Iraq), in 2013, to mention a few.

Although Arabism and pan-Arab, particularly in the 1950s and 1960s, was a popular model for Arabs, it did not prosper because of the interference of global and regional powers and the lack of both democratic systems and effective policies (Cohen 2014). While supporting MENA despotic regimes, the West (the United States and the G-7+1) attempted to impose, from the top down, the initiative of the "Greater Middle East," aimed at political democratization of the MENA region stretching from Morocco to Pakistan (Wittes 2004). According to the initiative, the region's key problem was defined not by the cultural (Arab) or religious (Islam) characteristics but by a lack of democracy (Stewart 2005).

Since 2011, the MENA region has experienced waves of protests and uprisings, known as the Arab Spring, in Tunisia, Egypt, Bahrain, Yemen, and Syria seeking democracy, fair economy, freedom, and social justice. Unfortunately, such events have politically divided MENA countries, turning people against each other, and have widened the differences among them. For example, Turkey and Qatar supported the uprisings by helping the newly elected governments that replaced the dictatorships, while Saudi Arabia and the UAE among other Gulf countries opposed the elected Islamic governments (dominated by the Muslim Brotherhood, al-Ikhwān al-Muslmīn) and saw them as a potential threat to their security (el-Aswad 2016a). In the meantime, the Shi'an uprising in Bahrain was quickly suppressed by the Gulf Cooperation Council's Peninsula Shield forces led by Saudi Arabia to prevent a similar uprising from spreading to neighboring GCC countries (el-Aswad 2016a). The political rivalry between Saudi Arabia and Iran for regional hegemony, coupled with sectarian conflicts, has further divided the region. It is very unfortunate that two of the richest countries in the MENA region are militarily battling each other in one of the poorest countries in that region, namely Yemen. Since March 2015, the UAE (and later Sudan) has joined Saudi Arabia in their war in Yemen. In addition to this internal malaise, Westerners, Europeans, and other foreign nationals have travelled to the region to fight for IS (Stern and Berger 2015).

The current conditions reflect the fragility and failure of authoritarian regimes to contain popular protests through peaceful political means. These political conditions add an element of uncertainty to the MENA region's economic environment, in particular, and well-being, in general. According to the 2015 final report of the United Nations High Commissioner for Refugees, 4.2 million Syrians are refugees, 6.5 million are displaced, 13.5 million need humanitarian assistance, 11 million require health assistance, 5.7 million children and adolescents are in need of educational assistance, and 2.4 million lack adequate shelters (United Nations High Commissioner for Refugees 2016). According to the United Nations Office for the Coordination of Humanitarian Affairs (2017), an estimated 17 million Yemeni people (60% of the total population) are food insecure whereas 7 million people are at risk of famine. And, an estimated 10.4 million Yemenis lack access to basic health care in addition to 2.9 million being either internally or externally displaced, often without legal papers of any type that confirm their citizenship and the like.

3.6.3 Militarization

Western and industrial countries have supplied economic and military aid to MENA countries, viewed as proxies in regional and global conflicts. Global powers, Arab-state forces, and non-state actors such as Al-Qa'ida, ISIS or IS (Da'ish), Al Nusra Front (*Jabhat al-Nusra*), and Hezbollah, among other parties and militias, rely heavily on arms to carry out their political agendas. Countries that have experienced civil war have recorded negative GDP growth. For instance, the GDP per capita of Syria decreased from $3555 in 2000 to $2441 in 2015 (United Nations Development Programme 2002, 2016b) (Tables 2.2 and 2.3). Libya, plagued with tribal militias, is struggling to retain a single government by building military arsenals.

The continued conflict in the MENA region involves armed struggle and motivates huge arms expenditures. Since the 1990s, the majority of MENA countries have been among the most heavily militarized in the world, reducing public spending on socioeconomic welfare, health care, and education. According to the *Global Firepower Index* (2017), the countries of the MENA region, high in military expenditures, ranked as follows: Saudi Arabia with $57 billion ranked 1 among MENA countries and 3 worldwide; Israel with $15.5 billion ranked 2 among MENA countries and 14 globally; the UAE with $14.5 billion ranked 3 among MENA countries and 16 globally; Algeria with $10.5 ranked 4 among MENA countries and 21 worldwide; and Turkey with $8.21 billion ranked 5 among MENA countries and 25 worldwide. Further, Oman, with $6.8 billion ranked 6 among MENA countries and 31 globally

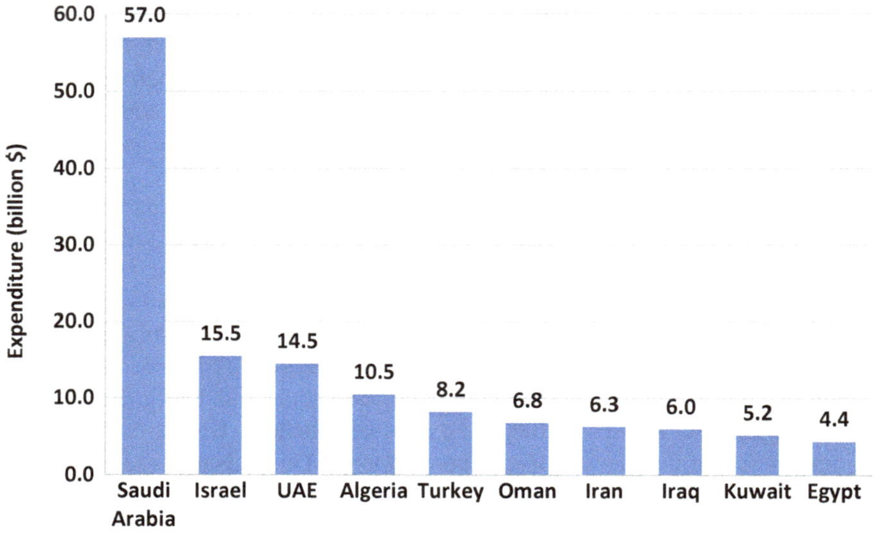

Fig. 3.4 Militarization in Middle East and North Africa region UAE = United Arab Emirates (Data from Global Firepower Index 2017; Bonn International Center for Conversion—Global Militarization Index—2017)

and Egypt, with $4.4 billion, ranked 10 among MENA countries and 45 worldwide (Fig. 3.4).

These rankings are consistent with the findings of the Global Militarization Index (Bonn International Center for Conversion 2017) that compares a country's military expenditure with its GDP and health expenditure. Scores used by the Global Militarization Index are based on the scale of 0–1.6 = very low; 1.6–3.2 = low; 3.2–4.8 = medium; 4.8–6.4 = high; 6.4–and above = very high (Bonn International Center for Conversion 2017). Most MENA countries are ranked high, with the exception of Saudi Arabia and Oman being ranked very high. According to *The Telegraph* (2017), "Qatar signs $12 billion deal to buy US fighter jets days after Trump accused it of sponsoring terrorism."

3.7 Quality of Life: Religion and Ideology

Religion is one of the most important factors for well-being, regardless of religious affiliation or service attendance (Graham and Crown 2014). The well-being benefits of religion appear to be associated with social activities and networking such as regular attendance at religious services (el-Aswad 2017; Huppert and Cooper 2014). Study findings indicate that people who are frequent attendees of worship places (church, mosque, or synagogue) have greater psychosocial well-being than those who are infrequent attendees (Bourne et al. 2015).

The MENA region is the cradle of monotheistic Abrahamic religions (Judaism, Christianity, and Islam) all of which have diverse and multiple sects and factions. Most of MENA countries constitute a Muslim-majority region in which most of the nation-states declare that Islam is their official religion (Pew Research Center 2017). According to the Pew Research Center, the largest religious group in the MENA region in 2010 was the Muslims, comprising 93%, whereas Christians made up roughly 4%, and the Jews, between 1 and 2% (Pew Research Center 2010).

This study proposes a distinction between ideology and religious worldviews. Although ideology implies certain economic and political orientations related particularly to power and authority, mostly as represented in the state or a particular group/party, religious worldview or cosmology indicates belief systems shared by a group of people or nation (el-Aswad 2002, 2003, 2016a, b). "Religious ideas about authority tend to follow from political ideas and political ideas often seek to ground themselves on religious thought" (Lee 2010: 14). Past and contemporary tragic events show that when religion is influenced by ideology, the outcome is a religious-political extremism and radicalism threatening people's well-being. For example, the Crusades in the 11th and 12th centuries were motivated by political ideology. In the 17th century, the politics of Georgian England was a branch of theology (Lee 2010) and the "Islamic ideology" is a force in modern Iranian politics (Lee 2010). By the same token, the Labor Zionists "sought to invoke Jewish values without reference to rabbinic Judaism or belief in God. The "New Jew" would be the product of collective political and social endeavor (Lee 2010). When the Egyptian government banned the Muslim Brotherhood as a terrorist organization on December 25, 2013, it politicized them (el-Aswad 2016b).

Religious extremism is considered a threat to well-being not only in Western countries, but also in all Muslim nations (el-Aswad 2013). More than 70% of Palestinian and Lebanese Muslims expressed their worry that violence might be carried out in their countries by Islamic extremists, as did Muslims in Egypt and Turkey (Pew Research Center 2011).

Islamist movements that apply the ideology of political Islam are not essentially strict religious groups concerned with issues of doctrine, beliefs and faith, but political organizations manipulating Islam as an ideological force to gain power over others or to resist power imposed on them. Using Islam as a power ideology is one of the major causes for the fragmentation and division that plague most of the MENA countries (el-Aswad 2016a). This situation is reflected in the Iran-Iraq War 1980–1988 (Sunni Vs. Shi'a) and Iraq's invasion of Kuwait 1990 (Sunni Vs. Sunni) as well as in the internal conflict in Libya, Yemen, civil war in Syria, and the boycott of Qatar by Saudi Arabia, the UAE, and Egypt in June 2017 (Salafi and Wahhabi Vs. both Muslim Brotherhood and Shi'a). It is to be noted here that, whereas both Sunni and Shi'a emphasize that the relationship between man and God is direct, the Shi'i doctrine of "spiritual leadership," or Imamate with specific reference to the Hidden Imam, constitutes a major difference (el-Aswad 2012).

It is worthy to note that believers in Abrahamic religions as well as adherents of sects within a particular religion co-exist in peace, but ideological and political differences and the lack of constructive dialogue result in grave conflict that negatively

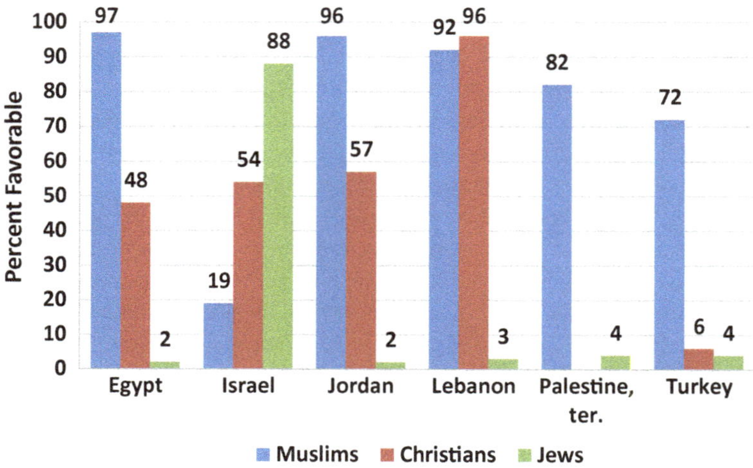

Fig. 3.5 How Muslims, Christians, and Jews view and rate each other. (Pew Research Center states that due to an administrative error, ratings of Christians in the Palestinian territories are not shown and in predominantly Muslim countries, figures are for Muslims only) (Data from Pew Research Center 2011)

affects the well-being of all inhabitants of the MENA region. According to the Pew Research Center (2011), Muslims' views toward Christians vary across countries. For example, in Egypt, which has a minority of Christian Copts, views are divided between a positive opinion with a rate of 48% and a negative opinion with a score of 47%. In Lebanon, which has a large Christian population, most of the Muslims express a positive view of Christians with a rate of 96%. Similarly, Jordan rates Christians positively, providing a score of 57%. Israel's view of Christians is slightly positive with a rate of 54%.

As shown in Fig. 3.5, Muslims' views toward the Jews are very low with negative ratings between 2% and 4%. Israel's views toward Muslims are also low with a rating of 19%. However, among Israel's minority Muslim community, views toward the Jews are divided between a positive opinion with a rate of 48% and a negative opinion with a rate of 49%.

3.8 Conclusion

Before addressing the quality of life in the MENA region, in this chapter I provided a broad account of the region's core geographic, demographic, and political features as well as the overall human development, particularly in the domains of economy, health, and education. This chapter has shown that the quality of life and well-being of MENA people have traversed through successive phases of progression and regression, triggered by external and internal factors, through various epochs of ancient, medieval, and modern history.

References

Abun-Nasr, J. (1987). *A history of the Maghrib in the Islamic period*. New York: Cambridge University Press.

Ballantyne, T., & Burton, A. (2012). *Empires and the reach of the global, 1870–1945*. Cambridge, MA: The Belknap Press of Harvard University Press.

Bonine, M., et al. (2011). *Is there a Middle East? The evolution of a geographical concept*. Palo Alto, CA: Stanford University Press.

Bonn International Center for Conversion. (2017). Global militarization index. Retrieved from http://gmi.bicc.de/index.php?page=gmi-new.

Bourne, P. A., Sharpe-Pryce, C., Francis, C., et al. (2015). The social psychology of religion and well-being: Is a belief in a God, good for one's well-being? An empirical inquiry. *Journal of Advanced Research in Psychology, 3*(1), 8–27.

Central Intelligence Agency. (2016). The world fact book. Washington, DC: Central Intelligence Agency. Retrieved from https://www.cia.gov/library/publications/the-world-factbook/geos/xx.html.

Chadwick, R. A. (2005). *First civilizations: Ancient Mesopotamia and ancient Egypt*. Oakville, CT: Equinox Publishing Ltd.

Cohen, S. A. (2014). *Future of the Middle East—United pan-Arab states: Divided by imperialism, united by destiny*. Bloomington, IN: AuthorHouse.

Commins, D. (2012). *The Gulf States: A modern history*. London: I. B. Tauris.

Daniel, M. H., & Tiberius, V. (2015). Well-being policy: What standard of well-being? *Journal of the American Philosophical Association*, Winter, 712–733. https://doi.org/10.1017/apa.2015.23.

Dawoody, A. (2015). *Public administration and policy in the Middle East*. New York: Springer.

Deaton, A. (2008). Income, health, and well-being around the world: Evidence from the Gallup World Poll. *Journal of Economic Perspectives, 22*(2), 53–72.

Derricourt, R. (2015). *Antiquity imagined: The remarkable legacy of Egypt and the ancient Near East*. London: I. B. Tauris.

Diener, E., Sandvik, E., Seidlitz, L., et al. (1993). The relationship between income and subjective well-being: Relative or absolute? *Social Indicators Research, 28*(3), 195–223.

Dirks, N. B. (1992). Introduction: Colonialism and culture. In N. B. Dirks (Ed.), *Colonialism and culture*. Ann Arbor, MI: University of Michigan Press.

el-Aswad, el-S. (1997). Archaic Egyptian cosmology. *Anthropos, 92*(1/3), 69–81.

el-Aswad, el-S. (2002). *Religion and folk cosmology: Scenarios of the visible and invisible in Rural Egypt*. Westport, CT: Praeger Press.

el-Aswad, el-S. (2003). Sanctified cosmology: Maintaining Muslim identity with globalism. *Journal of Social Affairs*, (20), 65–94.

el-Aswad, el-S. (2006). The permeability of the Middle East: The predicament of regional and global forces. *Digest of Middle East Studies* (DOMES), *15*(1), 113–120.

el-Aswad, el-S. (2012). *Muslim worldviews and everyday lives*. Lanham, MD: Alta Mira Press, Rowman & Littlefield Publisher.

el-Aswad, el-S. (2013). Images of Muslims in western scholarship and media after 9/11. *Digest of Middle East Studies* (DOMES), *22*(1), 39–56. https://doi.org/10.1111/dome.12010.

el-Aswad, el-S. (2016a). Political challenges confronting the Islamic world. In H. Tiliouine & R. J. Estes (Eds.), *The state of social progress of Islamic societies: Social, economic, political, and ideological challenges* (pp. 361–377). Cham, Switzerland: Springer International Publishing. https://doi.org/10.1007/978-3-319-24774-8_16.

el-Aswad, el-S. (2016b). State, nation and Islamism in contemporary Egypt: An anthropological perspective. *Urban Anthropology, 45*(1–2), 63–92.

el-Aswad, el-S. (2017). Empathy and emerging worldviews. In D. A. Leeming (Ed.), *Encyclopedia of Psychology and Religion* (pp. 1–4). New York, NY: Springer.

Ellison, C. W., & Smith, J. (1991). Toward an integrative measure of health and well-being. *Journal of Psychology and Theology, 19*(1), 35–45.

Estes, R. J. (2017). The search for well-being: From ancient to modern times. In R. J. Estes & M. J. Sirgy (Eds.), *The pursuit of human well-being: The untold global history* (pp. 1–30). Dordrecht, NL: Springer.
Estes, R. J., & Sirgy, M. J. (2017). *The pursuit of human well-being: The untold global history*. Dordrecht, NL: Springer.
Estes, R. J., & Sirgy, M. J. (2018). *Advances in well-being: Towards a better world*. London, New York: Rowman & Littlefield International.
Estes, R. J., & Tiliouine, H. (2014). Islamic development trends: From collective wishes to concerted actions. *Social Indicators Research, 116*(1), 67–114.
Estes, R. J., & Zhou, H. (2015). A conceptual approach to creating public-private partnerships in social welfare. *International Journal of Social Welfare, 24*(4), 348–363.
Fowden, G. (2013). *Before and after Muhammad: The first millennium refocused*. Princeton, NJ: Princeton University Press.
Freedom House. (2017). Freedom in the world 2017. Washington, DC: Freedom House. https://freedomhouse.org/sites/default/files/FH_FIW_2017_Report_Final.pdf.
Global Firepower Index. (2017). Defense spending by country. http://www.globalfirepower.com/defense-spending-budget.asp.
Graham, C., & Crown, S. (2014). Religion and well-being around the world: Social purpose, social time, or social insurance? *International Journal of Well-being, 4*(1), 1–27.
Gutas, D. (1998). *Greek thought, Arabic culture. The Graeco-Arabic translation movement in Baghdad and Early 'Abbasid Society*. London: Routledge.
Hamann, T., & Rosen, L. (2011). What makes the anthropology of educational policy implementation "anthropological"? In B. Levinson & M. Pollock (Eds.), *A companion to the anthropology of education* (pp. 461–477). New York: Wiley Blackwell.
Hersch, G. (2016). *Measuring well-being for public policy: Doing without theory* (Ph.D. thesis). University of California, San Diego. Retrieved from https://escholarship.org/uc/item/42c4b7f5.
Huppert, F. A., & Cooper, C. L. (2014). *Interventions and policies to enhance wellbeing: A complete reference guide* (Vol. VI). Chichester, West Sussex: Wiley.
Issawi, C. (1982). *An economic history of the Middle East and North Africa*. New York, NY: Columbia University Press.
Jawad, R. (2015, May 19–20). *Social protection and social policy systems in the MENA Region: Emerging Trends*. New York: United Nations Department of Economic and Social Affairs.
Karshenas M., & Moghadam, V. M. (2009). Bringing social policy back in: a look at the Middle East and North Africa. *International Journal of Social Welfare, 18*(s1), S52–S61.
Keddie, N. (1973). Is there a Middle East? *International Journal of Middle East Studies, 4*, 255–271.
Keulertz, M., et al. (2016). Material factors for the MENA Region: Data sources, trends and drivers. *Middle East and North Africa Regional Architecture*. Retrieved from https://www.cidob.org/content/download/65695/2014964/version/12/file/MENARA%20Concep%20paper%203_16.pdf.
Kwon, H. J. (2005). *The developmental welfare state and policy reforms in East Asia*. Basingstoke, UK: Palgrave-Macmillan.
Lammy, D., & Tyler, B. C. (2014). Wellbeing in four policy areas: Report by the all-party parliamentary group on wellbeing economics. Retrieved from http://b.3cdn.net/nefoundation/ccdf9782b6d8700f7c_lcm6i2ed7.pdf.
Lee, R. D. (2010). *Religion and Politics in the Middle East: Identity, Ideology, Institutions, and Attitudes*. Boulder, CO: Westview Press.
Maddison, A. (2003). *The world economy: Historical statistics*. Paris, France: Development Centre of the Organization for Economic Co-operation and Development.
Maddison, A. (2007). *Contours of the world economy 1-2030 AD: Essays in macro-economic history*. Oxford, UK: Oxford University Press.
Maisels, C. K. (1993). *The emergence of civilization: From hunting and gathering to agriculture, cities, and the state of the Near East*. London/New York: Routledge.
McDougall, J. (2011). The British and French Empires in the Arab World: Some problems of colonial state-formation and its legacy. In S. N. Cummings & R. Honeybunch (Eds.), *Sovereignty after*

Empire: Comparing the Middle East and Central Asia (pp. 44–66). Edinburgh, UK: Edinburgh University Press.
Michalos, A. (2014). *Encyclopedia of well-being and quality of life research (12 volumes)*. Dordrecht, NL: Springer.
O'Donnell, G., et al. (2014). *Wellbeing and Policy*. [Technical report]. London: Legatum Institute. Retrieved from https://li.com/docs/default-source/commission-on-wellbeing-and-policy/commission-on-wellbeing-and-policy-report—march-2014-pdf.pdf.
Organization for Economic Co-operation and Development. (2016). *Middle East and North Africa*. Retrieved from http://www.oecd.org/mena/Active_with_MENA_EN.pdf.
Orlin, L. L. (2007). *Life and thought in the Ancient Near East*. Ann Arbor, MI: University of Michigan Press.
Pappe, I. (2018). *Israel's new law is a form of apartheid*. Retrieved from https://www.thehindu.com/opinion/op-ed/israels-new-law-is-a-form-of-apartheid/article24513993.ece.
Peter, F., & Machin, D. (2015). *Quality of life*. Hoboken, NJ: Wiley.
Pew Research Center. (2010), *Middle East and North Africa: Global religious futures*. Washington, DC: Pew Research Center: Retrieved from http://www.globalreligiousfutures.org/regions/middle-east-north-africa.
Pew Research Center. (2011). Muslim-Western tensions persist. Retrieved from http://www.pewglobal.org/2011/07/21/muslim-western-tensions-persist/.
Pew Research Center. (2017). Many countries favor specific religions, officially or unofficially. Retrieved from http://www.pewforum.org/2017/10/03/many-countries-favor-specific-religions-officially-or-unofficially/.
Quirke, S. (2015). *Exploring religion in Ancient Egypt*. Malden, MA: Wiley.
Renima, A., Tiliouine, H., & Estes, R. J. (2016). The Islamic golden age: A story of the triumph of the Islamic civilization. In H. Tiliouine & R. J. Estes (Eds.), *The state of social progress of Islamic societies: Social, economic, political, and ideological challenges* (pp. 25–52). Cham, Switzerland: Springer International Publishing.
Richman, J. (2018). *Israel's new nationality law sparks immediate debate from American Jewish groups*. Retrieved from https://www.jns.org/israels-new-nationality-law-sparks-immediate-debate-from-american-jewish-groups/.
Schneer, J. (2010). *The Balfour declaration: The origins of the Arab-Israeli conflict*. New York: Random House.
Shapira, A. (2012). *Israel: A history*. Waltham, MA: Brandeis University Press.
Silva, J., Levin, V., & Morgand, M. (2012). *The way forward for social safety nets in the Middle East and North Africa*. Washington DC: World Bank.
Sirgy, M. J., Estes, R. J., & Selian, A. N. (2017). How we measure well-being: The data behind the history of well-being. In R. J. Estes & M. J. Sirgy (Eds.), *The pursuit of human well-being: The untold global history* (pp. 135–160). Dordrecht, NL: Springer.
Stern, J., & Berger, J. M. (2015). *ISIS: The State of Terror*. New York, NY: Ecco Press, an imprint of HarperCollins Publishers.
Stewart, D. J. (2005). The greater Middle East and reform in the Bush administration's ideological imagination. *Geographical Review, 95*(3), 400–424.
Suleiman, Y. (2013). Introduction. In Y. Suleiman (Ed.), *Language and identity in the Middle East and North Africa* (pp. 1–10). London, New York: Routledge.
Svara, J. (2015). *The ethics primer for public administration in government and nonprofit organizations*. Burlington, MA: Jones & Bartlett.
The Guardian. (2011). Qatar admits sending hundreds of troops to support Libya rebels. Retrieved from https://www.theguardian.com/world/2011/oct/26/qatar-troops-libya-rebels-support.
The Telegraph. (2017, June 15). Qatar signs $12bn deal to buy US fighter jets days after Trump accused it of sponsoring terrorism. Retrieved from http://www.telegraph.co.uk/news/2017/06/15/qatar-signs-12-billion-deal-buy-fighter-jets-us-frayed-diplomatic/.
Thompson, D. L. (1983). Public-private policy: An introduction. *Policy Study Journal, 11*(3), 365–562.

Tiliouine, H., & Estes, R. J. (2016). Social development in North African countries: Achievements and current challenges. In H. Tiliouine & R. J. Estes (Eds.), *The state of social progress of Islamic societies: Social, economic, political, and ideological challenges* (pp. 109–136). Dordrecht, NL: Springer.

Tiliouine, H., & Meziane, M. (2017). The history of well-being in the Middle East and North Africa (MENA). In R. J. Estes & M. J. Sirgy (Eds.), *The pursuit of human well-being: The untold global history* (pp. 523–563). Dordrecht, NL: Springer.

United Arab Emirates Government. (2018). *Social welfare programmes*. Retrieved from https://government.ae/en/information-and-services/social-affairs/social-welfare-programmes and https://www.abudhabi.ae/portal/public/en/citizens/benefits-for-nationals/social-support/social-welfare?_afrLoop=10769898005710168.

United Nations Development Programme. (2002). *Human development report 2002: Deepening democracy in a fragmented world.* Retrieved from http://hdr.undp.org/sites/default/files/reports/263/hdr_2002_en_complete.pdf.

United Nations Development Programme. (2003). *Human development report: 2003: Millennium Development Goals: A compact among nations to end human poverty.* Retrieved from http://hdr.undp.org/sites/default/files/reports/264/hdr_2003_en_complete.pdf.

United Nations Development Programme. (2016a). Human development reports. Human Development Index. Retrieved from http://hdr.undp.org/en/content/human-development-index-hdi.

United Nations Development Programme. (2016b). Human development reports: Human development index. Retrieved from http://hdr.undp.org/en/indicators/137506 and http://hdr.undp.org/sites/default/files/hdr2016_technical_notes.pdf.

United Nations High Commissioner for Refugees. (2016). *Protecting and supporting the displaced in Syria: End of year report 2015.* Damascus, Syria: United Nations High Commissioner for Refugees. Retrieved from http://www.unhcr.org/en-us/news/editorial/2016/2/56cad5a99/unhcr-syria-2015-end-of-year-report.html?query=Syria.

United Nations Office for the Coordination of Humanitarian Affairs. (2017). *Yemen.* Retrieved from https://www.unocha.org/yemen.

Wittes, T. C. (2004). The new U.S. proposal for a greater Middle East initiative: An evaluation. Washington, DC: The Brookings Institution. Retrieved from https://www.brookings.edu/research/the-new-u-s-proposal-for-a-greater-middle-east-initiative-an-evaluation/.

World Energy Council. (2016). *World energy resources*. Retrieved from https://www.worldenergy.org/wp-content/uploads/2016/10/World-Energy-Resources_Report_2016.pdf.

World Health Organization. (2017). World Health Statistics 2017. Monitoring health for the SDGs, Sustainable Development Goals. Retrieved from http://apps.who.int/iris/bitstream/10665/255336/1/9789241565486-eng.pdf?ua=1.

Wren-Lewis, S. (2013). Well-being as a primary good: Towards legitimate well-being policy. *Philosophy and Public Policy Quarterly, 31,* 2–9.

Chapter 4
Indicators of Quality of Life and Well-Being in the Middle East and North African Region: A Comparative Analysis

Abstract For analytic and comparative purposes, this chapter focuses on quality of life and well-being issues in selected countries of the Middle East and North Africa, namely Egypt, Iran, Israel, Tunisia, Turkey, and the United Arab Emirates. The study utilizes multiple objective and subjective outcome indicators to assess multiple dimensions of well-being including health, education, economy, and happiness. Further, this chapter includes a comparative analysis focusing on indicators of equity and inequality in differing domains of human development and well-being or ill-being. Finally, this study concludes that, despite the variations in quality of life across the Middle East and North Africa region, there is a common pattern of well-being related mainly to the progress made in the multiple dimensions of people's lives.

Keywords Quality of life · Well-being · Indicators · MENA region

4.1 Introduction

This chapter does not presume to cover the breadth and complexity of the topics required when addressing quality of life, social progress, and well-being in all Middle East and North African (MENA) countries. Rather, mentioned in previous chapters, for analytic and comparative purposes, this study focuses on six countries, Egypt, Iran, Israel, Tunisia, Turkey, and the United Arab Emirates (UAE). A thorough, yet concise study of quality of life and well-being requires a brief description of each of these selected states.

Determining whether human well-being or quality of life has improved over time is of crucial importance (McGillivray and Clarke 2007). However, an all-embracing study of quality of life and well-being of the MENA region must include indicators showing not only the improvement of quality of life but also its regression and the state of ill-being (Sirgy et al. 2017). This study, by focusing on these economically and demographically diverse countries, seeks to analyze and compare core features

el-S. el-Aswad, *The Quality of Life and Policy Issues among the Middle East and North African Countries*, Human Well-Being Research and Policy Making,
https://doi.org/10.1007/978-3-030-00326-5_4

and indicators of quality of life and human development at national, regional, and international levels between the years 1990 and 2015.

To secure a full understanding of people's quality of life, this study pays attention to both objective and subjective output indicators of well-being. Objective outcome indicators refer to objective information collected by government and non-governmental agencies focusing "*on capturing the state of well-being of individuals in the context of their communities*" (Sirgy et al. 2017: 137; italics are in the original). Outcome indicators measure and assess to what extent immediate objectives in health (measured, for instance, by life expectancy and infant and maternal mortality rates), education (measured by years of schooling, adult literacy, and enrollment rates) and economic standard of life (measured by gross domestic product [GDP] per capita) are achieved. Subjective indicators refer to people's states of subjective well-being (SWB) such as happiness, life satisfaction, and absence of ill-being. Overall, however, an emphasis is placed on "an integrated judgment of the person's life" (Diener 1984: 544). For instance, scholars maintain that there is a relationship between education and SWB, but this relationship is mediated by other elements such as health, income, and social mobility (Clifton 2017; Haybron and Tiberius 2015; Huppert and Cooper 2014; Lin 2016).

4.2 Quality of Life in the Middle East and North Africa

The following sections address well-being in each of the selected MENA countries and seek to determine their respective patterns of quality of life. The study then compares the indicators of quality of life among the selected countries.

4.2.1 Quality of Life in Egypt

Despite the political turmoil and economic hardships that Egyptians have experienced, particularly since 2011, there has been progress in some measures of their quality of life. The Human Development Index (HDI) value of Egypt improved from 0.547 in 1990 to 0.691 in 2015, an increase of 26.4%, situating the country in the medium category of human development with a rank of 111 out of 188 countries and territories. Figure 4.1 shows indicators of human development and well-being achieved by Egypt along with the dimensions of health, education, income, and demography between 1990 and 2015.

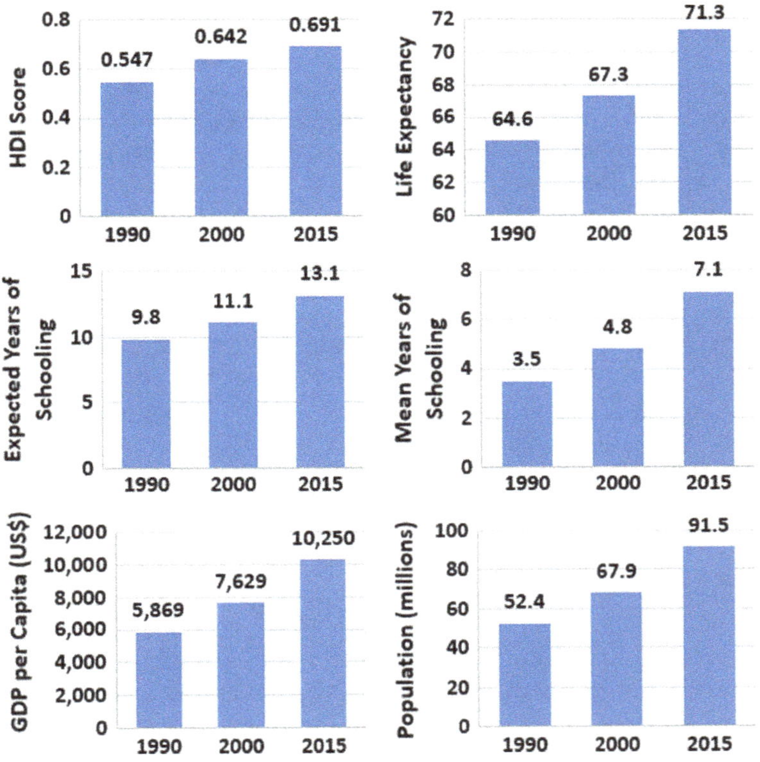

Fig. 4.1 Human Development Index of Egypt, 1990–2015. (Data from the Human Development Report [United Nations Development Programme 1992, 2016b])

4.2.1.1 Health and Well-Being

The third objective of the United Nations' Sustainable Development Goals is to "ensure healthy lives and promote well-being for all at all ages" (United Nations 2018).

Overall health outcomes within a given country are affected by factors such as institutional and medical care facilities, activities and programs, as well as other health indicators. As mentioned previously, health outcomes may include information about life expectancy, infant and maternal mortality rates, the number of live births, and communicable and non-communicable diseases (Sirgy et al. 2017).

Overall health outcomes in Egypt have significantly improved. In 1990, the indicator of life expectancy at birth in Egypt was 64.6 years; in 2015, it reached 71.3 years, having increased by 6.7 years (United Nations Development Programme 2016a, b) (Fig. 4.1). Although the indicator of life expectancy at birth in Egypt is lower than those of the other selected MENA countries, it is very close to the global life expectancy at birth of 71.4 years as measured in 2015 (World Health Organization 2018).

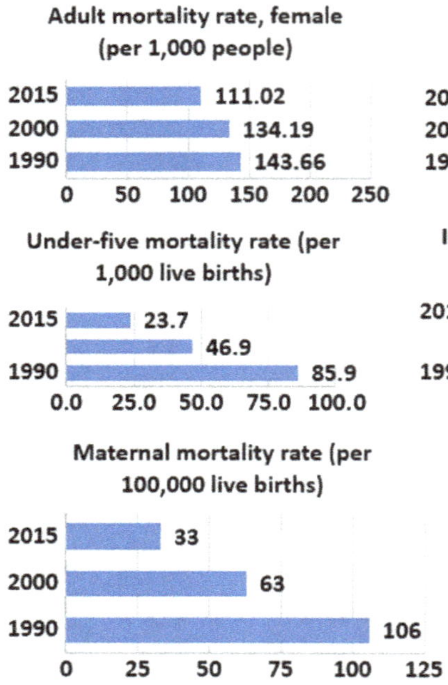

Fig. 4.2 Indicators of health in Egypt, 1990–2015. (Data from the Human Development Report [United Nations Development Programme 2002, 2016b] and World Health Organization [2016a, 2017])

The level of adult mortality is an important indicator for the comprehensive assessment of the mortality pattern in a population. The adult mortality rate for the female population in Egypt was reduced from 143.66 per 1000 people in 1990 to 134.19 per 1000 people in 2000, and then to 111.02 per 1000 people in 2015 (United Nations Development Programme 2002, 2016b; World Health Organization 2016a). The adult mortality rate for the male population decreased from 230.85 per 1000 people in 1990 to 216.86 per 1000 people in 2000, and then to 188.04 per 1000 people in 2015. The median adult mortality rate for the combined male and female population in Egypt was 151 per 1000 people, slightly above the global rate of adult mortality that reached 149 per 1000 population in 2015 (World Health Organization 2017). Likewise, the infant mortality rate was reduced from 63.37 per 1000 live births in 1990 to 37.30 per 1000 live births in 2000, and then to 20.10 per 1000 live births in 2015. The under-five mortality rate was also reduced from 85.90 per 1000 live births in 1990 to 46.90 per 1000 live births in 2000, and then to 23.70 per 1000 live births in 2015 (United Nations Development Programme 2016a; World Health Organization 2016a) (Fig. 4.2).

Figure 4.2 shows that the maternal mortality rate decreased from 106.63 per 100,000 live births in 1990 to 63 per 100,000 live births in 2000 and then to 33 per 100,000 live births in 2015, with an annual reduction of 4.5%. Although HIV prevalence among adults in Egypt (ages 15–49) "increased ten-fold between 2006 and 2010", it decreased to less than 0.1% (United Nations Development Programme 2016a), rendering Egypt a low-HIV-prevalence country.

According to the Institute for Health Metrics and Evaluation, the most prevalent causes of death in Egypt in 2015 included non-communicable diseases such as diabetes (53.8%), Alzheimer disease (30.4%), ischemic heart disease (28.1%), cirrhosis hepatitis C (19.2%), and cerebrovascular disease (12.2%). Deaths caused by communicable diseases such as lower respiratory tract infections were reduced to −37.8% of the total population. Deaths caused by life style behavior reached 38.8% due to alcohol and drug use and 20.5% due to consumption of tobacco. Deaths caused by environmental and occupational risk constituted 12.9% of the population (Institute for Health Metrics and Evaluation 2016a).

4.2.1.2 Education

The fourth objective of the United Nations' Sustainable Development Goals is to "ensure inclusive and equitable quality education and promote life-long learning opportunities for all" (United Nations 2018). Great emphasis has been put on education, particularly state-sponsored education, as an essential drive for development and quality of life in Egypt UNICEF (2015). The number of primary school students more than doubled in Egypt during the decade following the 1952 revolution. Whereas educational expansion in North Africa began in the 1960s, it began to expand in the Arabian Gulf countries in the 1970s (Eickelman 1992).

Overall, Egypt has shown significant progress in the domain of education. According to the HDI (UNESCO 2015; United Nations Development Programme 2016a), expected years of schooling in Egypt increased by 3.3 years between 1990 and 2015, when it increased from 9.8 years to 13.1 years, respectively. The indicator of the mean years of schooling in Egypt also improved and more than doubled from 1990, when it was 3.5 years, to 2015, when it became 7.1 years; this is an increase of 3.6 years. The adult literacy rate among those aged 15 years and older increased from 44.42% in 1986 to 75.2% in 2015 (UNESCO 2018a; United Nations Development Programme 2016a). Generally, the percentage of population, aged 25 and older, with at least some secondary education measured 61.4% in 2015 (UNESCO 2016; United Nations Development Programme 2016a).

The gross enrollment ratio of preprimary children increased from 21.32% in 2008 to 30% in 2015. The enrollment of students at primary and secondary schools was relatively high. For example, the gross enrollment ratio of the primary school-age population increased from 93% in 2011 to 104% in 2015. By the same token, the gross enrollment ratio of the secondary school-age population increased from 66.36% in 2009 to 86% in 2015. The gross enrollment ratio of university and tertiary level education grew from 28.88% in 2009 to 35.13% in 2015 (UNESCO 2018a; United Nations Development Programme 2016a). Mass higher education, mass communication, and new media have enabled people of the Middle East, particularly women, to participate in public space and political activities, practices almost unimagined in the past (el-Aswad 2014; Eickelman 2008, 2017).

According to the Social Progress Index (2017), Egypt scored very high (4 out of 6) and ranked 13 out of 101 countries in the percentage of students enrolled in globally ranked universities. Egypt also ranked high in number of globally ranked universities (Social Progress Index 2017).

4.2.1.3 Economic Well-Being

Egypt's economic well-being has been affected by the political and economic transformations (from feudalist, to socialist, to capitalist systems) that have occurred in its modern history (el-Aswad 2016a, 2016b). Tourism, agriculture, the Suez Canal, remittances, and the oil and gas industry are important sources of income for Egyptians. Economic well-being in Egypt tends not to be stable; rather, it fluctuates from year to year. For instance, the GDP per capita slowly but steadily improved by about 71.5% when it increased from $5869 in 1990 to $10,250 in 2015, which was lower than the average GDP per capita of $14,600 worldwide (United Nations Development Programme 2016b). The GDP in 2015 was $938 billion.

Ownership of decent housing is a key material element in securing well-being. According to the Social Progress Index (2017), Egypt underperformed on the indicator of availability of affordable housing, scoring 27.96 out of 100, with a rank of 120 out of 128 countries.

Regarding gender issues, it is to be noted that in Egypt, as in Iran, Turkey, Morocco, and elsewhere in the Middle East, informal economic roles of women have a greater impact on changing accepted gender roles in the public sphere than does formal legislation (Eickelman 2008).

4.2.1.4 Subjective Well-Being

According to the Organization for Economic Co-operation and Development (2013: 29), SWB is broadly defined as, "Good mental states, including all of the various evaluations, positive and negative, that people make of their lives, and the affective reactions of people to their experiences." Subjective well-being refers to the way people experience their lives, which may bear a strong or a weak relationship to the objective indicators of people's well-being (Huppert and Cooper 2014). Subjective indicators refer to people's states of well-being such as personal happiness, life satisfaction, and absence of ill-being. For example, the recurrence of public smiling in a country is sometimes used as an alternative indicator of the degree of subjective happiness and life satisfaction as well as well-being experienced by people (McGillivray and Clarke 2007; Sirgy et al. 2017).

According to the *World Database of Happiness* (Veenhoven 2017) that examined "average happiness" in 158 countries between 2005 and 2014, Egypt's average happiness was 5.5 out of 10 (10 = highest), indicating that Egypt's score of happiness made inclusion into the "above medium" category.

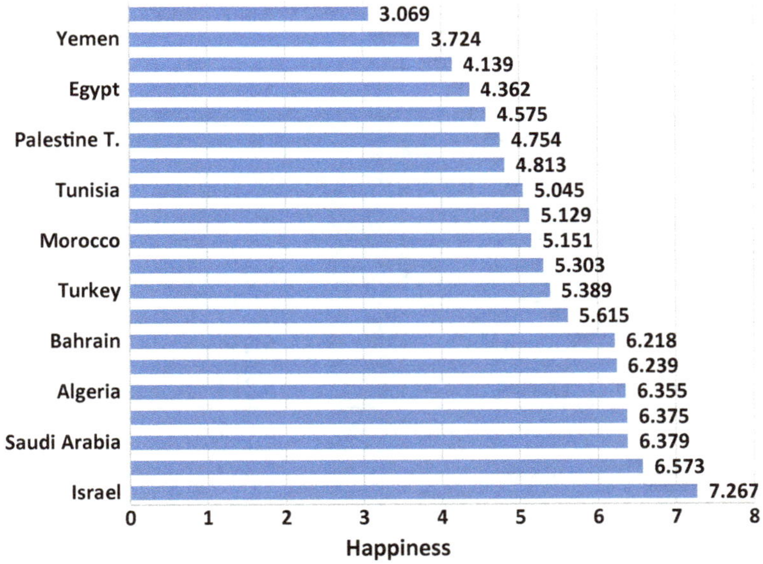

Fig. 4.3 Ranking of happiness in the Middle Eastern and North Africa region, 2015. (Data from the Human Development Report 2016 [United Nations Development Programme 2016b])

Since 2012, on March 20, the International Day of Happiness, the United Nations has released a "World Happiness Report" annually, in which nations are ranked according to the grades provided by their respondents. There are six variables upon which scores are evaluated. Two of the six variables relate to objective indicators, mainly GDP per capita and life expectancy at birth. The other four variables relate to SWB, including social support, and focus on indicators such as the help provided by relatives or friends in times of trouble, freedom to make life choices, generosity as measured by donations to charity, and freedom from corruption.

According to the World Happiness Report 2016 Update (Helliwell et al. 2016), Egypt scored 4.362 in 2015 (a slight decrease from previous years) and ranked 120 globally and 17 among MENA countries (Table 4.1 and Fig. 4.3). Figure 4.4 shows the happiness index among the selected MENA countries. The United Nations' World Happiness Report of 2017 indicated that Egypt's score of happiness in 2016 was 4.735, slightly higher than that of 2015 (Helliwell et al. 2017) (Table 4.2). In 2016, Egypt was globally ranked 104 (compared to the rank of 120 in 2015, and 14 among MENA countries (compared to the rank of 17 in 2015) (Table 4.2). The five top-ranking countries in the World Happiness Report 2016 were Norway (7.537), Denmark (7.522), Iceland (7.504), Switzerland (7.494), and Finland (7.469).

The social support indicator as assessed by the World Happiness Report refers to the help offered by a relative or friend to a person/respondent in a situation of crisis or troubles. The score Egyptians obtained was very low and should be higher when considering that Egyptians have been described in terms of their social capital or

Table 4.1 Ranking of Happiness in the MENA region, 2015 (Data extracted from World Happiness Report [Helliwell et al. 2016])

	Rank	Country	Score
1	11	Israel	7.267
2	28	UAE	6.573
3	34	Saudi Arabia	6.379
4	36	Qatar	6.375
5	38	Algeria	6.355
6	41	Kuwait	6.239
7	42	Bahrain	6.218
8	67	Libya	5.615
9	78	Turkey	5.389
10	80	Jordan	5.303
11	90	Morocco	5.151
12	93	Lebanon	5.129
13	98	Tunisia	5.045
14	105	Iran	4.813
15	108	Palestine T.	4.754
16	112	Iraq	4.575
17	120	Egypt	4.362
18	133	Sudan	4.139
19	147	Yemen	3.724
20	156	Syria	3.069
NA	NA	Oman	NA

Nations are ranked depending on the average grades provided by the respondents.

"relatedness," which "is of fundamental significance in Egyptian culture" (el-Aswad 1999: 432). And "social capital (or 'relatedness') is more significantly related to subjective well-being than economic indicators" (Sirgy 2011: 5). Egyptians, particularly the poor, "assert that it is not the material accumulation, but the *baraka* (blessing) of what they have that matters" (el-Aswad 2002: 47). The value of blessing is related to Egyptians' concept of *as-satr*, which implies such multiple meanings as those indicating whatever can be protected, guarded, covered, and secured (el-Aswad 2012). These multiple meanings encompass economic, social, personal, spiritual, and cosmological dimensions that can be called "cosmic capital." There is not a minimum or

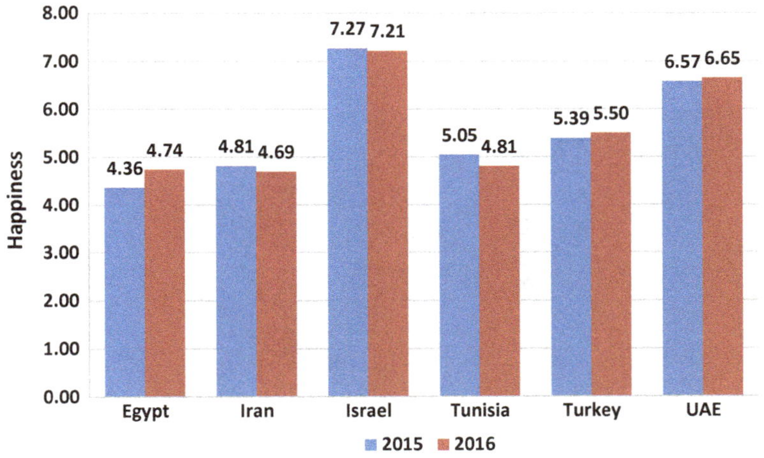

Fig. 4.4 Happiness in selected countries of the Middle East and North Africa, 2015–2016. (Data from the World Happiness Report [Helliwell et al. 2016])

maximum economic standard against which the state of *as-satr* or cosmic capital is measured. If someone is asked about her/his financial condition, he or she is expected to respond, "'It is secured (covered) and praise be to Allah'. This may explain the Egyptians' unusual ability to smile cheerfully and spontaneously as well as to be receptive to jokes and humor while experiencing unbearable economic hardships" (el-Aswad 2002: 48). "[I]t is the pursuit of happiness rather than of economic wealth that is the driving force underlying the high degree of positive 'happy' behavior seen in developing countries" (Sirgy et al. 2017: 140–141).

Humor and jokes play an important role in Egyptian lives, especially during stressful and troubling circumstances. Egyptians manipulate jokes as a social mechanism of expression against state repression and global aggression (el-Aswad 1990, 1993, 2004). When Egyptians tell a joke, they want not merely to amuse people, but also to make themselves laugh. Laughter shows a desire to live. Egyptians use humor to express their own viewpoint and/or to cope with their problems (El-Menawy 2017).

4.2.2 *Quality of Life in the Islamic Republic of Iran*

There has been progressive development in the Islamic Republic of Iran over the past 25 years. Iran improved its HDI value from 0.572 in 1990 to 0.774 in 2015, an increase of 35.3%. Iran achieved a high human development category, ranking 69 worldwide out of 188 countries and territories. Figure 4.5 shows the indicators of human development and well-being in the dimensions of health, education, income, and demography in Iran between 1990 and 2015. Increases have been made across all dimensions.

Table 4.2 Ranking of Happiness in the MENA region, 2016 (Data from World Happiness Report [Helliwell et al. 2016])

	Rank	Country	Score
1	11	Israel	7.213
2	21	UAE	6.648
3	34	Qatar	6.403
4	37	Saudi Arabia	6.344
5	39	Kuwait	6.105
6	41	Bahrain	6.087
7	53	Algeria	5.872
8	68	Libya	5.569
9	69	Turkey	5.5
10	74	Jordan	5.336
11	84	Morocco	5.235
12	88	Lebanon	5.225
13	102	Tunisia	4.805
14	104	Egypt	4.735
15	108	Iran	4.692
16	117	Iraq	4.497
17	130	Sudan	4.139
18	146	Yemen	3.593
19	152	Syria	3.462
NA	NA	Palestine T.	NA
NA	NA	Oman	NA

Nations are ranked depending on the average grades provided by the respondents.

4.2.2.1 Health Well-Being

The indicator of life expectancy at birth in Iran increased by 11.8 years between 1990 when it was 63.8 years and 2015 when it reached 75.6 years (Fig. 4.6). As a further positive indicator of health well-being, the adult female mortality rate has steadily deceased over the past 25 years: In 1990 it measured 184.49 per 1000 people; in 2000 it was 126.13 per 1000 people (World Health Organization 2016b), and in 2015 it was 64 per 1000 people. Globally, the overall adult mortality rate was 149 per 1000 population in 2015 (World Health Organization 2017). The adult male mortality rate also decreased from 278.97 per 1000 people in 1990 to 177.08 per 1000 people in 2000 (World Health Organization 2016b) and then to 105 per 1000 people in 2015. Similarly, the under-five mortality rate was reduced from 56.70 live births in 1990 to 34.30 per 1000 live births in 2000, and then to 15.5 per 1000 live births in 2015. The infant mortality rate decreased from 44.10 per 1000 live births in 1990 to 36 per 1000 live births in 2000 and then to 13.4 per 1000 live births in 2015. The maternal mortality rate also decreased from 123 per 100,000 live births in 1990 to

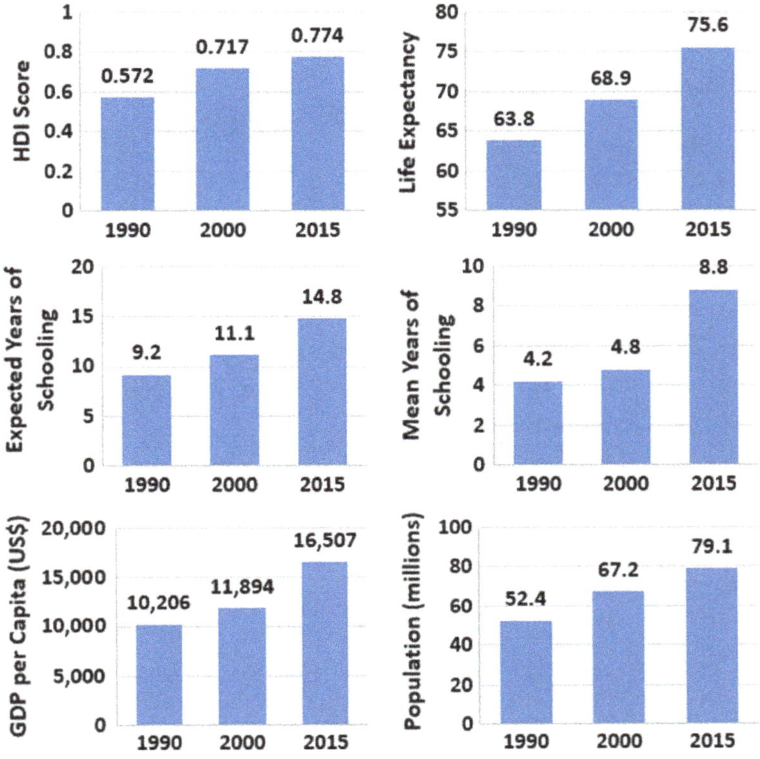

Fig. 4.5 Human Development Index of Iran, 1990–2015. (Data from the Human Development Report [United Nations Development Programme 1992, 2016b])

51 per 100,000 live births in 2000 and then to 25 per 100,000 live births in 2015 (United Nations Development Programme 2016b; World Health Organization 2016b) (Fig. 4.6). Furthermore, HIV prevalence was reduced from 0.2% in 2005 to 0.1% for adults (ages 15–49) (UNICEF 2006; United Nations Development Programme 2016a).

According to the Institute for Health Metrics and Evaluation (2016b), the causes of premature death in Iran by non-communicable diseases included diabetes (67.2%), hypertensive heart disease (23.2%), stomach cancer (17.5%), and ischemic heart disease (4.3%). Causes of premature death due to communicable diseases included tuberculosis (3.5 per 100,000 people) (United Nations Development Programme 2016) and lower respiratory infection (−31.0%). Behavioral risks included consumption of tobacco (12.7%) and alcohol and drug use (4.8%). Causes of death due to environmental and occupational factors were recorded at 8.7% (Institute for Health Metrics and Evaluation 2016b).

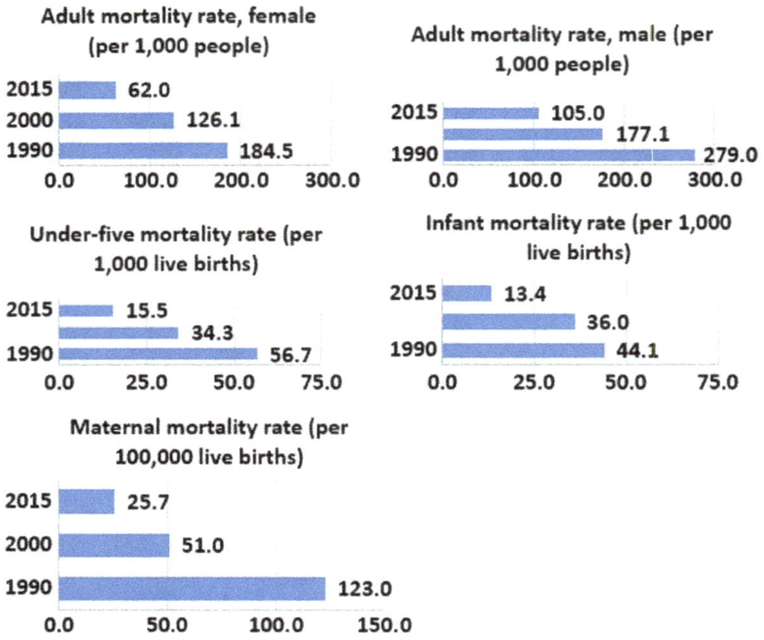

Fig. 4.6 Health well-being in Iran, 1990–2015. (Data from the Human Development Report [United Nations Development Programme 2016a] and the World Health Organization, 2016a, 2017)

4.2.2.2 Education

Iran's expected years of schooling increased by 5.6 years between 1990 and 2015. Expected years of schooling were 9.2 years in 1990 and increased to 14.8 years by 2015. Similarly, the calculated mean for years of schooling increased by 4.6 years. The mean for years spent in school in 1990 was 4.2 years, but it more than doubled by 2015 when it reached 8.8 years. Other positive indicators showing progress in education in Iran include an increase in the adult literacy rate for people aged 15 and older from 65.53% in 1991 to 86.8% in 2015. The gross enrollment ratio for preprimary (preschool aged) children also increased from in 41.31% in 2010 to 50.59% in 2015, whereas the gross enrollment ratio for the primary (school aged) children improved from 105 to 109% of the population in 2015 (UNESCO 2018b; United Nations Development Programme 2016a).

The gross enrollment ratio for the secondary school-aged population grew from 77.18% in 2010 to 88% in 2015, very close to that of Egypt in 2015 (86%). The percentage of population aged 25 and older with at least some secondary education in Iran in 2015 was 67.7%, slightly higher than that in Egypt (61.4%). In addition, the gross enrollment ratio of the tertiary school-aged population in Iran increased from 36% in 2009 to 71% in 2015 (UNESCO 2018b; United Nations Development Programme 2016a).

4.2.2.3 Economic Well-Being

Iran's economy is based on oil or hydrocarbon sectors, agricultural sectors, and service sectors. However, economic activity and government revenues depend to a large extent on oil revenues. Currently, Iran ranks second in the world in natural gas reserves and fourth in proven crude oil reserves (World Bank 2018a).

The GDP per capita of Iran increased by about 60.6% between 1990, when it was $10,206, and 2015, when it reached $16,507, which was $1907 higher than the average GDP per capita of $14,600 worldwide. The total GDP was $1289.9 billion. Exports and imports comprised 43.1% of the total GDP. Iran's average annual growth was about 2.7% in 2015, higher than the average worldwide annual growth of 2.3% (United Nations Development Programme 2016a).

Poverty is estimated to have fallen from 8.1% in 2009 to 3.7% in 2015. The population living below the income poverty line of $1.90 a day was 0.1% (United Nations Development Programme 2016a). The current account surplus is estimated to have increased to 6.5% of the GDP in 2016, up from 2.7% in 2015, benefiting strongly from the removal of oil sanctions and a recovery in exports (World Bank 2018a).

As indicated by the Social Progress Index (2016), Iran underperformed on the indicator of availability of affordable housing, scoring 31.58 out of 100 with a rank of 113 out of 128 countries.

4.2.2.4 Subjective Well-Being

People who feel socially integrated and are close to and receiving comfort and support from others in their community are content and happy (Keyes 1998). However, the history of the level of happiness in Iran has shown a continuous regression in both rank and score. According to the World Database of Happiness (Veenhoven 2017), Iran's happiness between 2005 and 2014 scored 5.8 out of 10. The World Happiness Report 2016 Update indicated that Iran attained a score of 4.813 in 2013–2015, ranked 105 globally (Helliwell et al. 2016) and 14 among MENA countries. In 2014–2016, Iran, with a score of 4.692, was less happy compared with 2014 (with a grade of 5.8) and 2015 (with a grade of 4.813), respectively. Also, Iran's rank decreased from 105 to 108 (out of 155 countries) at the global level (Helliwell et al. 2017) and from 14 to 15 at the regional level (Fig. 4.7).

4.2.3 Quality of Life in Israel

Israel's HDI value was 0.785 in 1990 and improved to 0.899 in 2015, evidencing an increase of 14.5%. The country achieved the category of "very high" human development and was ranked 19 out of 188 countries and territories. Figure 4.8

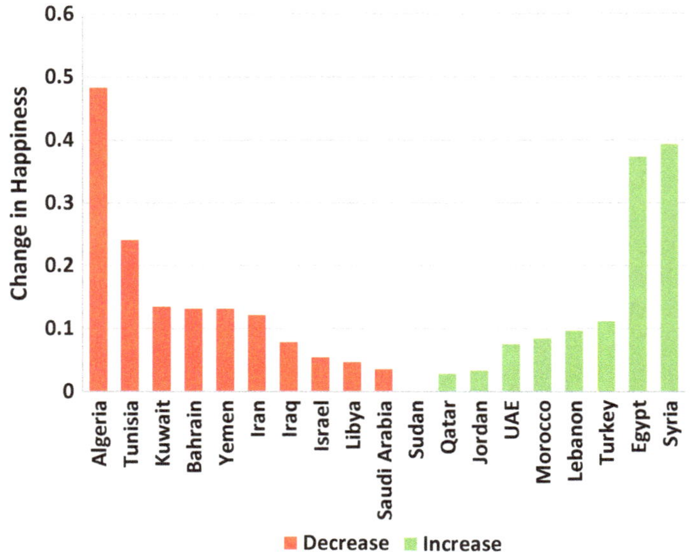

Fig. 4.7 Change in happiness between 2015 and 2016 UAE = United Arab Emirates. (Data from the Human Development Report 2016 [United Nations Development Programme 2016b])

shows the outcome indicators of human development and well-being achieved by Israel in the dimensions of health, education, income, population, and demography between 1990 and 2015.

4.2.3.1 Health Well-Being

The indicator of life expectancy at birth in Israel increased by 6.2 years in the span of 25 years. In 1990, life expectancy was 76.4 years of age and by 2015 it had increased to 82.6 (United Nations Development Programme 2016a) (Fig. 4.9). As a further positive indicator of health well-being, the adult female mortality rate deceased steadily over the past 24 years: In 1990 it measured 70.60 per 1000 people, in 2000 it was 54.71 per 1000 people, and then in 2014 it measured 48.98 per 1000 people. The adult male mortality rate also declined from 107.04 per 1000 people in 1990 to 102.58 per 1000 people in 2000 and then to 72.23 per 1000 people in 2014. Furthermore, the under-five mortality rate decreased from 11.60 per 1000 live births in 1990 to 6.90 per 1000 live births, then to 3.80 per 1000 live births in 2014. The infant mortality rate was also reduced from 9.70 per 1000 live births in 1990 to 5.60 per 1000 live births in 2000 and then to 3.2 per 1000 live births in 2015. In addition, the maternal mortality rate decreased from 11 per 100,000 live births in 1990 to 8 per 100,000 live births in 2000, and then to 5 per 100,000 live births in 2014 (United Nations Development Programme 2016a; World Health Organization 2016c). The HIV prevalence was also reduced in Israel from 40.8 per 1000 people in 1990, to

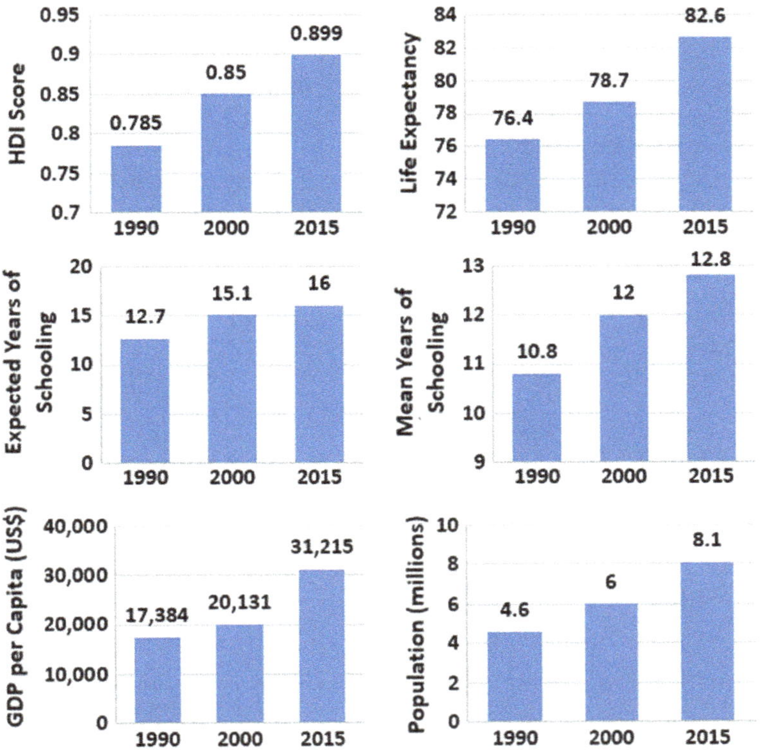

Fig. 4.8 Human Development Index of Israel, 1990–2015. (Data from the Human Development Report [United Nations Development Programme 1992, 2016b])

16.2 per 1000 people in 2000, to 10.8 per 1000 people in 2010, and then to 6.7 per 1000 people in 2012 (UNICEF 2013). Even with these significant reductions, Israel ranks highest among the MENA countries in HIV prevalence.

According to the Institute for Health Metrics and Evaluation (2016c), the causes of death in Israel of non-communicable diseases included lung cancer (22.7%), cerebrovascular disease (7.8%), diabetes (1.2%), ischemic heart disease (0.8%), and tuberculosis (0.2 per 100,000 people). Causes of death of communicable diseases included lower respiratory infections (49.9%). Causes of death of behavioral risk included alcohol and drug use (23.3%) and tobacco use (3.6%). Also quantified were deaths due to factors of occupational risks (24.4%) and environmental/air pollution (7.3%). Poor objective health and disability are associated with lower ratings in subjective well-being (Huppert and Cooper 2014).

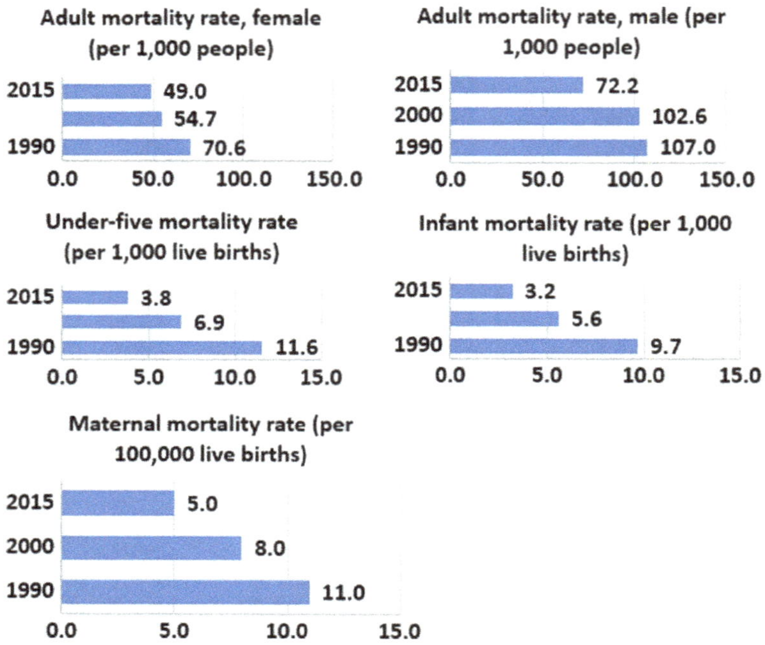

Fig. 4.9 Health well-being in Israel, 1990–2015. (Data from the Human Development Report [United Nations Development Programme 2016b] and the World Health Organization, 2016c, 2017)

4.2.3.2 Education

The indicator of expected years of schooling in Israel increased 3.3 years from 12.7 years in 1990 to 16.0 years in 2015, whereas the indicator of mean years of schooling increased by 2.0 years, from 10.8 years in 1990 to 12.8 years in 2015 (United Nations Development Programme 2016a). The adult literacy rate of people aged 15 and older improved from 91.75% in 1983 to 98.7% in 2016 (Central Intelligence Agency 2018). Comparatively, the gross enrollment ratio of preprimary education students increased from 92.28% in 2010 to 53% in 2015. Similarly, the gross enrollment ratio of primary education students grew from 97.04% (of the primary school-aged population) in 2010 to 104.49% in 2015. The gross enrollment ratio of secondary education students also improved from 98.04% (of the secondary school-aged population) in 2010 to 102.84% in 2015 (Fig. 4.8). The gross enrollment ratio of the tertiary education students increased from 59.76% (of the tertiary school-aged population) in 2008 to 64.75% in 2015 (UNESCO 2018c; UNICEF (2013; United Nations Development Programme 2016a), less than that of Iran (71%).

4.2.3.3 Economic Well-Being

Israel's economy is characterized by advanced industry and high-technology military equipment, oil products, natural gas, and cut diamonds. Israel's GDP per capita improved; it was $17,384 in 1990 and reached $31,215 in 2015 (Fig. 4.8). Israel's GDP in 2015 was $265.4 billion (United Nations Development Programme 2016b).

According to the Central Intelligence Agency (2018), the total growth of the GDP reduced to an average of roughly 2.6% per year during the period 2014–2016 due to decreased investment and slow domestic and international demand caused by Israel's uncertain security situation in the region. However, the percentage of population living below the income poverty line of $1.90 a day was 0.3% in 2007–2010 and increased to 0.7% in 2012 (World Bank 2018b).

Concerning the indicator of the availability of affordable housing, Israel, according to Social Progress Index (2017), scored very low (26.32 out of 100), ranking 111 out of 128 countries.

4.2.3.4 Subjective Well-Being

According to the World Database of Happiness (Veenhoven 2017), Israel achieved a high score of 7.3 out of 10 between 2005 and 2014. The World Happiness Report 2016 Update (Helliwell et al. 2016) stated that in 2013–2015, Israel achieved a grade of 7.267, ranked 11 globally (Helliwell et al. 2016) and rated first among MENA countries (Table 4.2). In 2014–2016, however, Israel, with a score of 7.213, was less happy compared with 2015 but kept its rank of 11 globally (Helliwell et al. 2017) and first regionally (Table 4.2). It is interesting to observe that Israel kept its global ranking of 11 for more than 7 years since the span of 2010–2012, when it had a score of 7.301 (Helliwell et al. 2013) (Fig. 4.7). Despite the advanced rank of Israel, a recent study, "Measuring and Assessing Well-Being in Israel" (OECD 2015), argued that Israel faces a problem related to the indicator of social support. To be more specific, this study stated that social connections are one of the areas where the evidence base for measuring well-being is weakest in Israel (OECD 2015). And "while Israeli tended to be very sociable, a comparatively large share of Israelis have no one to count on for help or talk to about personal matters" (OECD 2015: 43).

4.2.4 Quality of Life in Tunisia

Tunisia's HDI score improved from 0.582 in 1990 to 0.725 in 2015. The country fell within the level of "high" human development with a rank 97 out of 188 countries and territories. Figure 4.10 shows that Tunisia secured positive human development and well-being in the domains of health, education, economy, and population during the period 1990–2015.

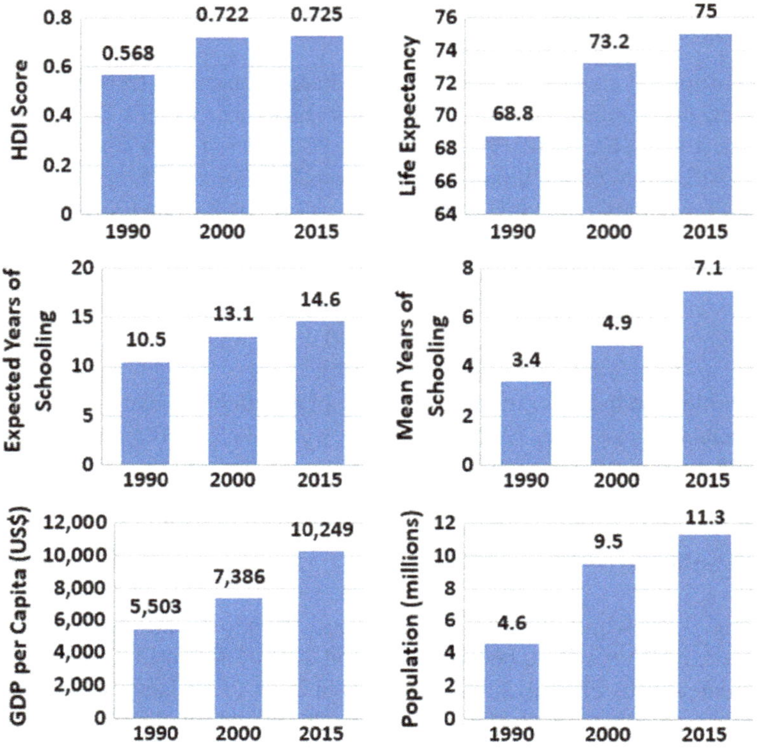

Fig. 4.10 Human Development Index of Tunisia, 1990–2015. (Data extracted from Human Development Report [United Nations Development Programme 1992, 2016b])

4.2.4.1 Health Well-Being

Tunisia's life expectancy at birth increased by 6.2 years between 1990 and 2015 when it improved, respectively, from 68.8 years to 75.0 years. In 2015, women's life expectancy at birth was 77.4 years, whereas that of men was 72.7 years. There is a reported 12.2% inequality in life expectancy rating in favor of women (United Nations Development Programme 2016a) (Fig. 4.11).

As further positive indicators of health well-being, the adult mortality rates (female and male) and both infant and under-five morality rates have steadily deceased over the past 25 years: The adult mortality rate of the female population was reduced from 137.31 per 1000 people in 1990 to 83.67 per 1000 people in 2000 and then to 70.65 per 1000 people in 2015. By the same token, the adult mortality rate of the male population dropped from 185.12 per 1000 people in 1990 to 140.14 per 1000 people in 2000 and then to 112.02 per 1000 people in 2015. Figure 4.11 shows that the infant mortality rate decreased from 40.2 per 1000 live births in 1990 to 13.30 per 1000 live births in 2000 and then to 10.90 per 1000 live births in 2015. The under-five mortality rate also diminished from 56.80 per 1000 live births in 1990 to 31.70 per

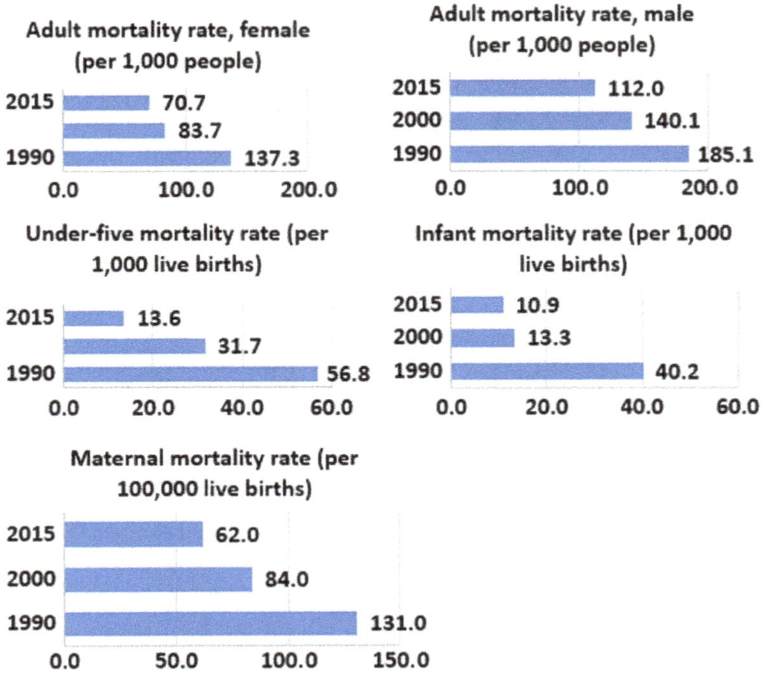

Fig. 4.11 Health well-being in Tunisia, 1990–2015. (Data from the Human Development Report [United Nations Development Programme 2016a; World Health Organization, 2016c, 2017])

1000 per live births in 2015. Moreover, the maternal mortality rate declined from 131 per 100,000 live births in 1990 to 84 per 100,000 live births in 2000 and then to 62 per 100,000 live births in 2015 (United Nations Development Programme 2016a; World Health Organization 2016d). The percentage of HIV prevalence among adult population (ages 15–49) was reduced from 0.2% in 2001 to 0.1% in 2016 (Central Intelligence Agency 2018; United Nations Development Programme 2016a).

According to the Institute for Health Metrics and Evaluation (2016d) the most prevalent causes of death in Tunisia included non-communicable diseases such as Alzheimer disease (51.8%), diabetes (51.6), ischemic heart disease (31.6%), cerebrovascular disease (23.6%), and lung cancer (39.3%). Death caused by communicable disease included lower respiratory infection (−9.0%) and tuberculosis (2 per 100,000 people). Death caused by risky behavior included use of tobacco (24.2%) and consumption of an unhealthy diet (17.1%). Deaths caused by environmental and air pollution were calculated at 20.7% whereas those attributed to occupational risks were calculated at 15.7%. A substantial amount of research has focused on perceived environmental problems, such as air pollution and noise, which are associated with lower subjective well-being (Huppert and Cooper 2014).

4.2.4.2 Education

High-quality education is a vital part of well-being. Tunisia's expected years of schooling increased by 4.1 years between 1990, when it was 10.5 years, and 2015 when it reached 14.6 years. Mean years of schooling increased by 3.7 years and developed from 3.4 years in 1990 to 7.1 years in 2015. However, mean years of schooling for the female population was 6.7 years; mean years of schooling for the male population was 7.8 years (Fig. 4.10).

The adult literacy rate (aged 15 and older) in Tunisia increased from 73.03% in 2004 to 81.8% in 2015 (UNESCO 2018d; United Nations Development Programme 2016a). The gross enrollment ratio of the preprimary population (preschool-age children) also grew from 41.32% in 2013 to 44.37% in 2016. The gross enrollment ratio of the primary school-aged population improved substantially from 104.09% in 2008 to 114.71% in 2016. Additionally, the gross enrollment ratio of the secondary school-aged population (secondary education students) changed from 90.41% in 2008 to 92.87% in 2016; the gross enrollment ratio of the tertiary school-aged population increased from 33.71 to 35% in 2015 (UNESCO 2018d; United Nations Development Programme 2016a) (Fig. 4.10).

4.2.4.3 Economic Well-Being

Tunisia has improved its economic well-being. For instance, Tunisia's GDP per capita increased by 86.2% between 1990, when it was \$5503, and 2015, when it reached \$10,249 (Fig. 4.10). Tunisia's total GDP in 2015 was \$119.1 billion (United Nations Development Programme 2016a; International Labor Organization 2017) and the inflation rate was about 4.9%. Two percent of the population were living below the income poverty line of \$1.90 a day. According to the Social Progress Index (2016), Tunisia underperformed on the indicator of availability of affordable housing, scoring 28.98 out of 100 with a rank of 118 out of 128 countries.

4.2.4.4 Subjective Well-Being

Happiness is considered as one of the indicators of SWB, which is essential in implementing policies aimed at improving the overall well-being of people. The rapid social and political changes occurring in Tunisia may explain the deterioration in its happiness levels. Between 2005 and 2014, according to the World Database of Happiness (Veenhoven 2017), Tunisia achieved a score of 5.5 out of 10. Despite the political tribulation of 2011, Tunisia managed to maintain a moderate level of happiness. In 2015, Tunisia achieved a score of 5.045 and ranked 98 worldwide (Helliwell et al. 2016) and 13 among MENA countries (Table 4.2). But, in 2016, a decrease in the level of happiness in Tunisia was reported and Tunisia, with a score of 4.805, moved down 4 places to a rank of 102 globally (Helliwell et al. 2017) but kept its rank of 13 regionally (Fig. 4.7).

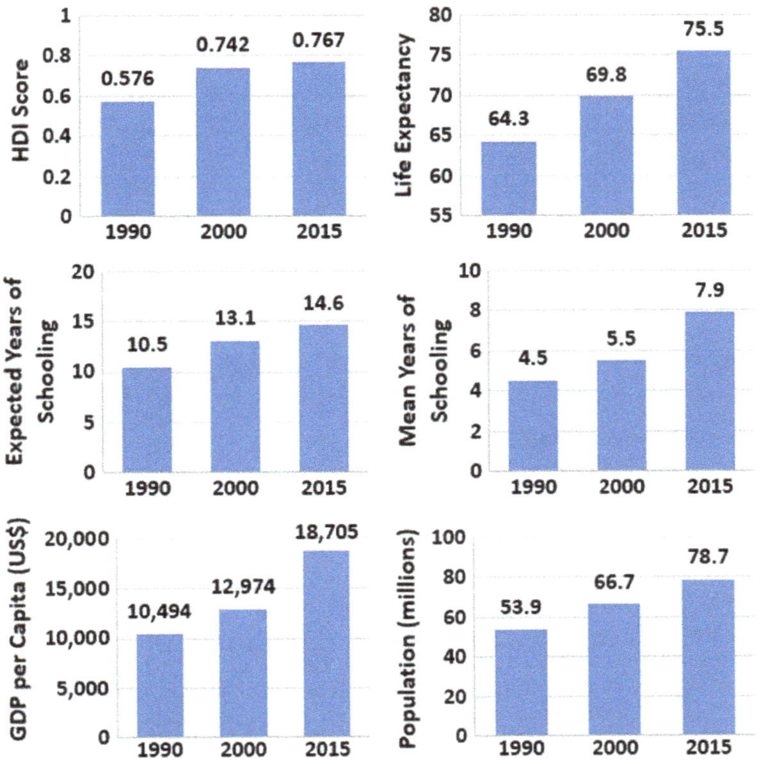

Fig. 4.12 Human Development Index of Turkey, 1990–2015. (Data from the Human Development Report [United Nations Development Programme 1992, 2016b])

4.2.5 Quality of Life in Turkey

Turkey's HDI value for 2015 was 0.767, which put the country in the high human development category and ranked it 71 out of 188 countries and territories. Turkey's HDI value increased from 0.576 in 1990 to 0.767 in 2015, an increase of 33.2%. As shown in Fig. 4.12, there is strong evidence for the development of human well-being in the domains of health, education, economy, and population during the period from 1990 to 2015.

4.2.5.1 Health and Well-Being

Health in Turkey is rated one of the highest among the six MENA countries.

Turkey's life expectancy at birth increased by 11.2 years in 25 years. It was 64.3 years in 1990 and advanced to 75.5 years in 2015 (Fig. 4.13). Other positive indicators of health well-being include the following: The adult female mortality rate

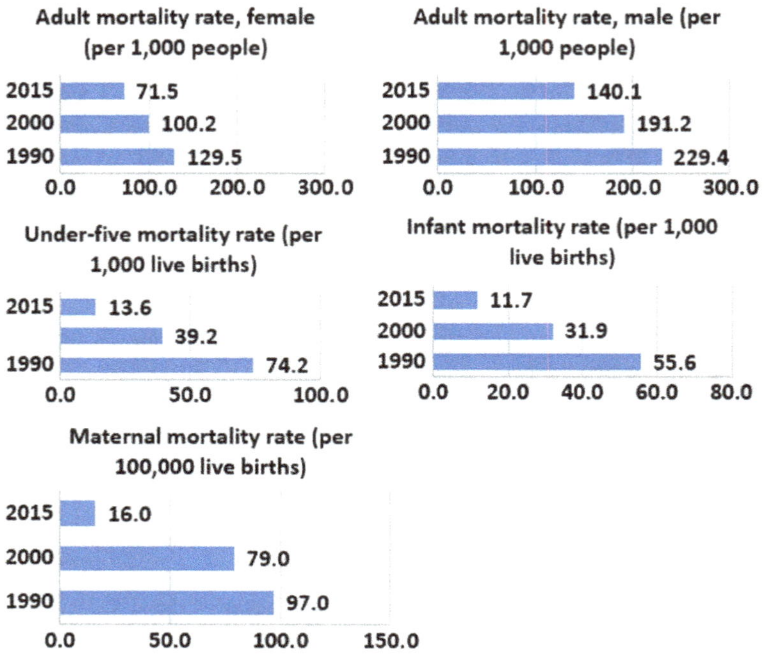

Fig. 4.13 Health well-being in Turkey, 1990–2015. (Data from the Human Development Report [United Nations Development Programme 2016a; World Health Organization, 2016e, 2017])

decreased from 129.46 per 1000 people in 1990 to 100.23 per 1000 people in 2000 and then to 71.53 per 1000 people in 2015, and the adult male mortality rate reduced from 229.40 per 1000 people in 1990 to 191.21 per 1000 people in 2000, and then to 140.12 per 1000 people in 2015. The under-five mortality rate declined from 74.20 per 1000 live births in 1990 to 39.20 per 1000 live births in 200 and then to 13.60 per 1000 live births in 2015. The infant mortality rate dropped from 55.60 per 1000 live births in 1990 to 31.90 per 1000 live births in 2000 and then to 11.70 per 1000 live births in 2015. Comparably, the maternal mortality rate decreased from 97 per 100,000 people in 1990 to 79 per 100,000 people in 2000 and then to 16 per 100,000 people in 2015 (UNESCO 2018e; United Nations Development Programme 2016a; World Health Organization 2016e) (Fig. 4.13).

According to the Institute for Health Metrics and Evaluation (2016e), causes of death in Turkey included non-communicable diseases such as ischemic heart disease (17.6%), cerebrovascular disease (23.6%), lung cancer (18.4%), Alzheimer disease (46.1%), hypertensive heart disease (41.4%), colorectal cancer (31.4%), and diabetes (28.0%).

Death caused by communicable disease included lower respiratory infections (−54.9%) and tuberculosis (0.6 per 100,000 people). Deaths caused by behavioral risk included consuming tobacco (4.1%). Neither alcohol consumption nor drugs were recorded as a cause of death. Deaths caused by environmental factors included air pollution (3.5%), whereas deaths caused by occupational risks were reported at 16.3%.

4.2.5.2 Education

Turkey's expected years of schooling increased by 5.7 years between 1990 and 2015 (Fig. 4.12). They increased from 8.9 years in 1990 to 14.6 years in 2015. The mean years of schooling increased by 3.4 years, improving from 4.5 years in 1990 to 7.9 years in 2015. The difference between expected years of schooling for men and women was not significant. Expected years of schooling for women were 14 years, whereas those for men were 15 years (United Nations Development Programme 2016a).

The adult literacy rate (for those aged 15 and older) advanced from 79.23% in 1990 to 95.6% in 2015. The gross enrollment ratio of preprimary education (of preschool-aged children) improved from 17.93% in 2008 to 29.23% in 2015. The gross enrollment ratio of primary education (of the primary school-aged population) developed from 100.1% in 2008 to 107% in 2015. The gross enrollment ratio of secondary education (of the secondary school-aged population) advanced from 80.02% in 2009 to 103.05% in 2015. The gross enrollment ratio of tertiary education (of the tertiary school-aged population) also increased from 40.22% in 2008 to 95.43% in 2015 (United Nations Development Programme 2016a) (Fig. 4.12).

4.2.5.3 Economic Well-Being

Turkey's economic performance has been progressive. Macroeconomic and fiscal stability were at the heart of its performance, enabling increased employment, incomes, and prosperity. Although Turkey remains highly dependent on imported oil and gas, the petrochemical, automotive, and electronics industries have risen in importance and surpassed other traditional sectors such as textiles and clothing within Turkey's export mix (Central Intelligence Agency 2018). Turkey's GDP per capita increased by 78.2% between 1990, when it was $10.49, to 2015 when it reached $18,705 (Fig. 4.12). Turkey's total GDP in 2015 was $1491.40 billion.

The incidence of poverty decreased significantly by 2015, and extreme poverty has fallen even faster. The population living below the income poverty line of $1.90 a day declined from 3.70% of the people in 2003 to 0.3% in 2015 (World Bank 2018c)

According to the Social Progress Index (2016), Turkey performed within expected ranges on the indicator of "availability of affordable housing," scoring 53.89 out of 100, achieving a ranking 40 out of 128 countries.

4.2.5.4 Subjective Well-Being

Although starting from a relatively middle base, Turkey is among the MENA countries where people have shown improvement in their life satisfaction and happiness. But, according to the World Database of Happiness (Veenhoven 2017), Turkey attained a moderate score of 6.0 out of 10 between 2005 and 2014. According to the World Happiness Report Update, in 2015, Turkey achieved a grade of 5.389, ranked 78 globally (Helliwell et al. 2016) and 9 among MENA states (Table 4.1). As shown in Table 4.2, in 2016, Turkey improved its level of happiness by a score of 5.500, gaining 9 places and moving up from the rank of 78 to the rank of 69 worldwide (Helliwell et al. 2017), while maintaining the rank of 9 among MENA countries (Fig. 4.7).

4.2.6 Quality of Life in the United Arab Emirates

The HDI value for the UAE improved from 0.726 in 1990 to 0.840 in 2015, with an increase of 15.7%, positioning it in the very high human development category with a rank of 42 out of 188 countries and territories (United Nations Development Programme 2016a). Figure 4.14 shows that the Emirates has achieved development of human well-being in the domains of health, education, economy, and population during the 25-year period from 1990 to 2015.

4.2.6.1 Health Well-Being

Life expectancy at birth in the UAE improved from 71.5 years in 1990 to 77.1 years in 2015, an increase of 5.6 years (Fig. 4.15). Other indicators showing the progress in health well-being in the UAE include the following: The adult female mortality rate decreased from 117.82 per 1000 people in 1990 to 85.94 per 1000 people in 2000 and to 56.64 per 1000 people in 2015. The adult male mortality rate also declined from 146.00 per 1000 people in 1990 to 111.57 per 1000 people in 2000 and then to 80.51 per 1000 people in 2015. Figure 4.15 shows that the under-five mortality rate shrunk from 16.60 per 1000 live births in 1990 to 11.20 per 1000 live births in 2000 and to 7.80 per 1000 live births in 2015. The infant mortality rate also decreased from 14.2 per 1000 live births in 1990 to 9.60 per 1000 live births in 2000 and then to 6.70 per 1000 live births in 2015. Similarly, the maternal mortality rate diminished from 17 per 100,000 people in 1990 to 8 per 100,000 people in 2000 and then to 6 per 100,000 people in 2015 (UNESCO 2018f; United Nations Development Programme 2016a; World Health Organization 2016f) (Fig. 4.15).

According to the Institute for Health Metrics and Evaluation (2016f), causes of death in the UAE included non-communicable diseases such as ischemic heart disease (215.2%), chronic obstructive pulmonary disease (178.8%), cerebrovascular disease (188.4%), and diabetes (219.9). Deaths of communicable disease have included

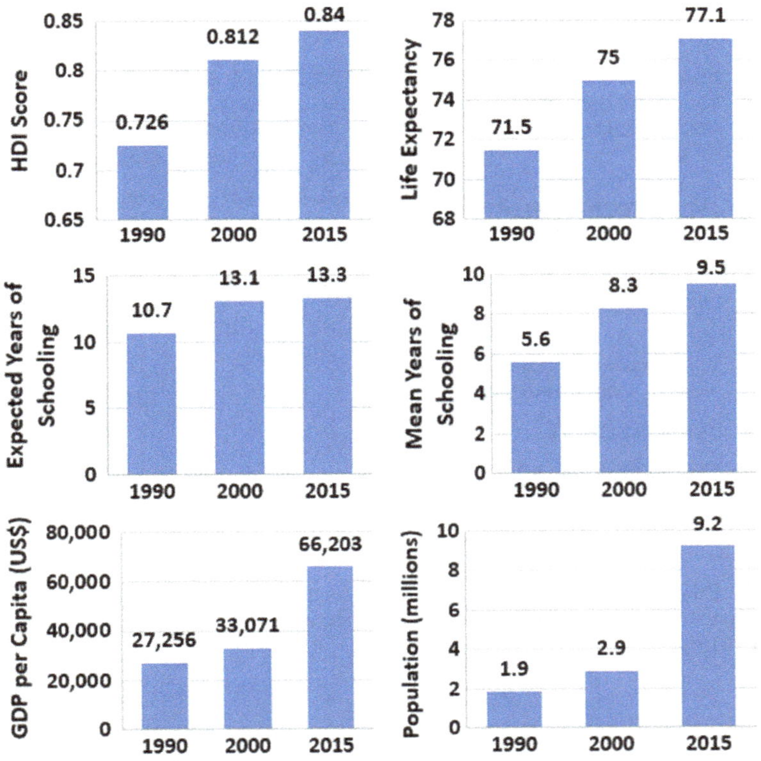

Fig. 4.14 Human Development Index of the United Arab Emirates, 1990–2015. (Data from the Human Development Report [United Nations Development Programme 1992, 2016b])

lower respiratory infections (−130.6%) and those of behavioral risk included tobacco (4.1%). Death has also been caused by environmental (3.5%) and occupational risk (16.3%) factors or risks.

4.2.6.2 Education

Expected years of schooling in the Emirates increased by 2.6 years over 25 years; it was 10.7 in 1990 and increased to 13.3 years in 2015 (Fig. 4.14). The mean years of schooling increased by 3.9 years from 5.6 years in 1990 to 9.5 years in 2015 (United Nations Development Programme 2016a). The expected years of schooling among the female population were higher than those of the male population. For example, the expected years of schooling for women in 2015 were 13.9 years, whereas those for men were 12.9 years.

The literacy rate for people (15 years and older) increased from 90.03% in 2005 to 93.8% in 2015. Notably, literacy rates were higher among women than men. In 2015, the literacy rate among women was 95.9%, whereas that for men it was

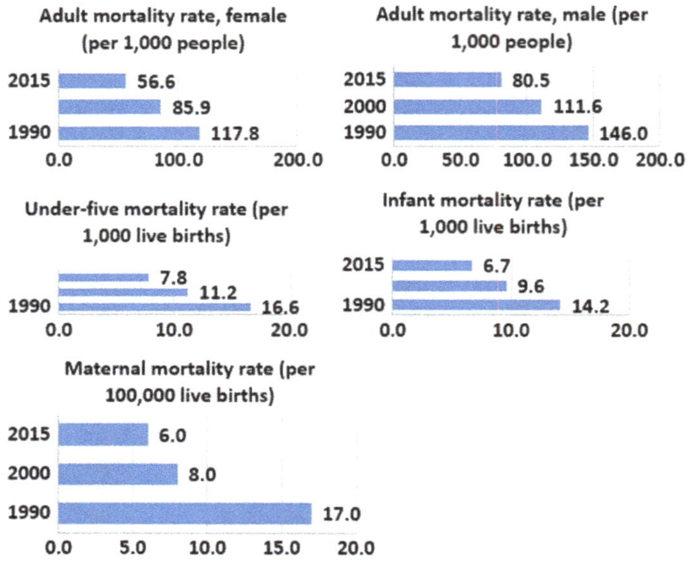

Fig. 4.15 Health well-being in the United Arab Emirates, 1990–2015. (Data from the Human Development Report [United Nations Development Programme 2016a] and the World Health Organization, 2016f, 2017)

93.1% (Central Intelligence Agency 2015). The gross enrollment ratio of preprimary education (or, of preschool-age children) improved from 63.7% in 2010 to 92% in 2015. Comparably, the gross enrollment ratio of primary education (of the primary school-age population) increased from 95.36% in 2009 to 116.35% in 2015. The gross enrollment ratio of secondary education grew from 62.24% in 1990 to 95.81% in 2016. The gross enrollment ratio of tertiary education students also increased from 6.53% in 1990 to 22% in 2015 (UNESCO 2018f; United Nations Development Programme 2016a).

4.2.6.3 Economic Well-Being

The GDP per capita in the UAE has fluctuated by about 36.7% in 25 years. It was $104,615 in 1990, reached $108,791 in 2000, but decreased to $66,203 in 2015 (United Nations Development Programme 2016a) (Fig. 4.14). However, the Emirates is among the world's wealthiest states. The total GDP in 2015 was calculated at $605.3 billion.

According to the Social Progress Index (2016), the UAE performed within expected ranges (but higher than Turkey) on the indicator of "availability of affordable housing," scoring 60.47 out of 100 with a rank of 23 out of 128 countries. Most houses provided to nationals in the Emirates are part of a state-sponsored housing initiative (el-Aswad 2016c: 195).

4.2.6.4 Subjective Well-Being

According to the World Database of Happiness (Veenhoven 2017), which examined happiness in 158 countries between 2005 and 2014, the UAE achieved a high score of 7.3 out of 10. The World Happiness Report 2016 Update (Helliwell et al. 2016) stated that in 2015 the UAE achieved a score of 6.573 out of 10, ranked 28 globally (out of 155 countries) and second among MENA countries (first among Arab states) (Table 4.1). In 2016, the level or score of happiness of the UAE increased from 6.573 to 6.648, moving up 7 places from the rank of 28 to 21 worldwide as well as maintaining its second-place rank among MENA countries and first place rank among Arab states (Table 4.2, Fig. 4.7). It is interesting to note that in February 2016, the UAE announced the appointment of a Minister of State for Happiness and Wellbeing in the new UAE Cabinet (UAE 2017). The new ministry aims to promote the UAE's plans and policies to promote happiness of the UAE society.

It is worth noting that the method used to divide the Emirati nationals from the expatriate population residing in the country reduced its actual score of happiness. Helliwell (2016: 23) and his team argued, "Splitting the UAE sample into two groups would give a 2013–2015 Emirati ladder average of 7.06 (ranking 15th), and non-Emirati average 6.48 (ranking 31st), very close to the overall average of 6.57 (ranking 28th)." However, such a method was not applied to other diverse and multiethnic states such as Israel and Turkey.

4.3 Comparative Analysis

To conduct a comparative analysis, the study focuses on the selected countries despite their differences in achievement on the HDI categories (very high, high, medium, and low). Out of the six countries, two countries, Israel and Emirates, were ranked in 2015 very high in human development with an HDI rank higher than 80 out of 100. Three countries, Iran Tunisia, and Turkey, were ranked high in human development with an HDI rank of 70–9. One country, Egypt, ranked within the medium human development category with an HDI rank of 55–69. However, because Egypt achieved an HDI rank of 69, which is close to the rank of 70 (high human development), it might be practical to include Egypt in the comparative analysis. The following sections deal with important indicators related to human rights, freedom of expression, and religious tolerance, among other indicators. In addition, one section addresses the indicators of equity and inequality between the selected MENA countries in the differing domains of human development and well-being.

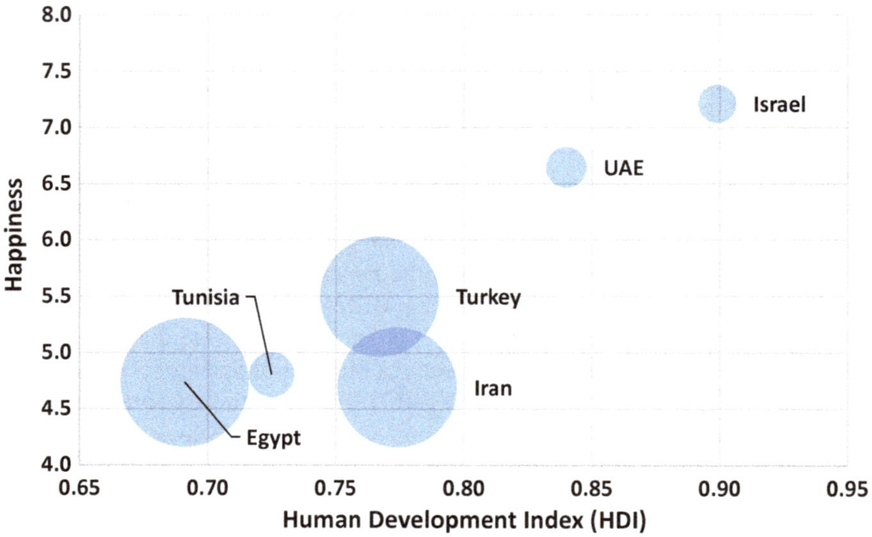

Fig. 4.16 Happiness and Human Development Index of selected countries of the Middle East and Northern Africa, 2015, UAE = United Arab Emirates. (Data from the Human Development Report 2016 [United Nations Development Programme 2016b])

4.3.1 Happiness and Human Development

This section deals with the relation between the indicator of "happiness" and overall HDI value of the selected MENA countries. For example, despite Iran's HDI value (0.774) being higher than that of Egypt (0.691), Tunisia (0.725), and Turkey (0.767) and despite the apparent economic advances made by Iran compared to Egypt (as shown in Fig. 4.16), it seems that Iranians were less happy than the populations of the other countries. As shown in Fig. 4.17, Iran's score of happiness in 2016 was 4.692, which was less than those of Egypt (4.735), Tunisia (4.805), and Turkey (5.500) (see Fig. 4.4). Iranian unhappiness has been expressed through antigovernment demonstrations, from December 2017 through January 2018, resulting from their fading expectations of a good economy and better life due to the lifting of sanctions following the 2015 nuclear treaty. The Iranian "citizens are not all poor, property-less, or uneducated, but they have been suffering from high youth unemployment, a housing market disfigured by speculation, relaxed labor regulations, and the general inability to live the life promised by their educational status or even to match their parents' standard of living" (Ehsani and Keshavarzian 2018: 5). In a comparable manner, antigovernment street protests erupted in Tunisia (in January 2018) due to political and economic problems including poverty and unemployment (Smith-Spark 2018). It is worth noting that the level of happiness in Iran and Tunisia has shown continuous regression in both global rank and score.

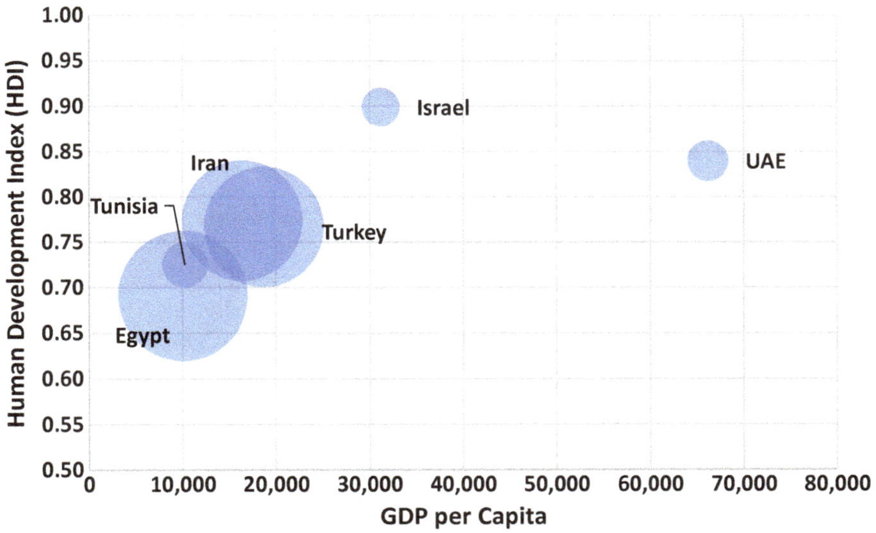

Fig. 4.17 Happiness and gross domestic product per capita in selected Middle Countries, 2015 UAE = United Arab Emirates. (Data from the Human Development Report 2016 [United Nations Development Programme 2016b])

4.3.2 Inequality Issues

This section tackles the problem of inequality in the selected MENA countries. "Society is considered just if two distinct principles are met. The first principle of a just society holds when there is equality in the assignment of basic rights and duties. The second principle of the just society holds when inequalities are justified to benefit the least advantaged members of the society" (Sirgy 2011: 11). However, the problem of inequality is not restricted to a specific country or region. Some "fundamentalist Christians and ultra-orthodox Jews exclude women from many aspects of public life, and in countries such as the United States, Russia, and Japan marked inequalities persist in some regions" (Eickelman 2008: 143).

It is worth noting that gender inequality is part of the Gender Development Index (GDI) created by the Human Development Report to specify a female to male ratio in the HDI. The GDI reflects gender disparity, taking into consideration inequality in favor of men or women in achievement along the dimensions of health, education, and income (United Nations Development Programme 2016a).

Inequality affects quality of life and well-being in all MENA countries. It cripples progress in health, education, income, and political participation. According to the HDR (United Nations Development Programme 2016a), the GDI reflects gender inequalities in achievement in the three dimensions of the HDI: health, "measured by female and male life expectancy at birth"; education, "measured by female and male expected years of schooling for children and mean years for adults aged 25 years and older"; and economic resources, "measured by female and male estimated GPD per capita." As inequality increases, loss in well-being and human development also increases. Although an overall high GDI value (Israel, UAE, Turkey, and Tunisia) indicates that the inequality between men and women is less than a low GDI value (Iran and Egypt), data show that there are differences in scores of indicators among the dimensions of health, education, and economy.

Concerning inequality in health issues in the MENA countries in 2015, Fig. 4.18 shows that the life expectancy at birth or the average age of women was higher than that of men, as is the case at the global level. However, there are disparities or differences between women and men among the selected countries. The following numbers indicate how much longer women live than their male counterparts: Turkey (8.85%), Tunisia (6.46%), Egypt (6.36%), Israel (4.21%), Iran (2.95%), and the UAE (2.61%).

For the indicator of "expected years of schooling," Fig. 4.18 shows that women in Israel, Tunisia, and UAE have achieved more years of education than men. In contrast, women in Egypt, Iran, and Turkey have achieved fewer years than men. For the indicator of "mean years of schooling," men have higher scores than women in four countries, namely Egypt, Iran, Tunisia, and Turkey. Only two countries, Israel and the UAE, have higher scores on the indicator of "mean years of schooling" for women than men. However, the difference between the females' score of 10.06 and males' score of 8.7, regarding "mean years of schooling" in the UAE is higher than the difference between females (12.8) and males (12.7) in Israel.

Recent research shows that although economic growth in the region has lifted many people out of poverty, the decline in poverty rates in the MENA region has occurred at a slower pace than in other regions, such as Eastern Europe and Central Asia or East Asia and the Pacific (Drine 2012). Two large groups of the population, children and rural residents, face a higher than average risk of poverty. They suffer from inequality of opportunities, which is aggravated by lack of access to social and economic services, resulting in lower human development outcomes (Silva et al. 2012).

When one looks at gender disparity in income, there is an obvious inequality between men and women in favor of men. Although the magnitude of the income disparity between men and women is lower in some countries, such as Israel, Turkey, the UAE, and Egypt, it is relatively high in other countries, such Iran and Tunisia. To be more specific, Israeli women make 59.4% as much as men; Turkish women make 39.4% as much as men; Emirati women make 33.9% as much as men; Egyptian women make 31.1% as much as men; Tunisian women make 29.2% as much as men; and Iranian women make 18.6% as much as men. In each case, men earn significantly more income than women. In only one country (Israel) do women earn more than 50% of what men earn. The rest earn less than half of what the men earn.

It must be noted that the Human Development Report (United Nations Development Programme 2016b) refers to inequality-adjusted HDI or IHDI, which takes into consideration inequality in all three dimensions of the HDI by omitting each dimension's average value based on its level of inequality. This means that IHDI is actually the HDI reduced due to inequalities. Put differently, the HDI may lose

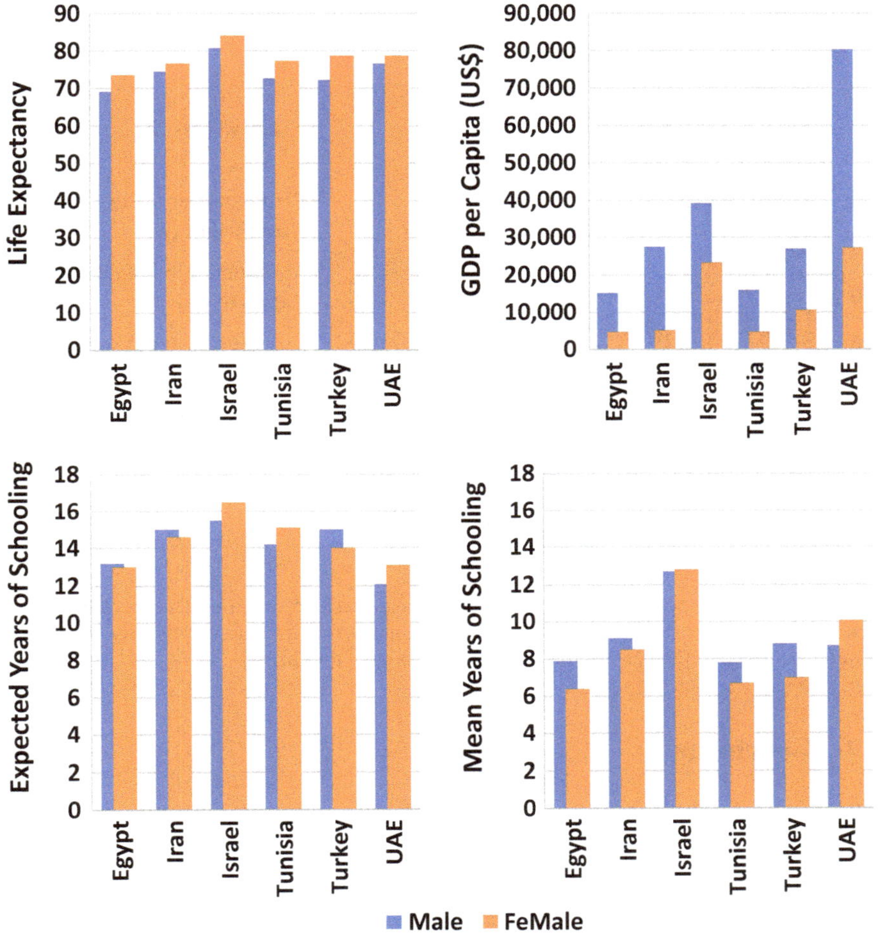

Fig. 4.18 Gender Development Index in the countries of the Middle East and North Africa. (Data from the Human Development Report [United Nations Development Programme 2016a])

value because of the negative impact of inequality. Consequently, there is a "loss" in human development generated by the difference between the HDI and the IHDI that can be displayed as a percentage. Based on this inequality criterion, MENA countries lose their HDI values. However, they differ in the overall "loss" based on the level of inequality attributed to each country. Table 4.2 and Fig. 4.19 show that Iran's overall loss (33.1%) is greater than those of other MENA countries such as Egypt (29.0%), Tunisia (22.5%), Turkey (15.9%), and Israel (13.5%).

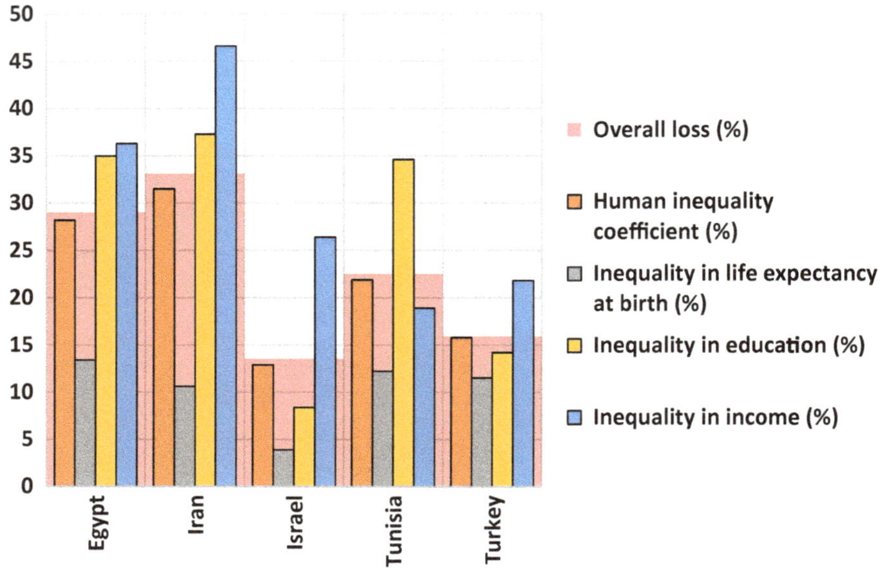

Fig. 4.19 Inequality-adjusted Human Development Indexes for 5 countries. Due to a lack of relevant data, the IHDI has not been calculated for the United Arab Emirates. (Data from the Human Development Report [United Nations Development Programme 2016a])

4.4 Conclusion

This chapter has reviewed the progress MENA countries have made over the past 25 years (1990–2015) in various dimensions of quality of life and well-being. This inquiry concludes that the selected MENA countries have made significant progress in almost all domains of well-being, notwithstanding the variations and differences in the outcomes among these countries. To be more specific, most MENA countries have achieved steady progress in HDI over the past 25 years. The progress is represented by increased life expectancy at birth, lower rates of maternal, child, and infant mortality, increased rates of literacy, partial economic growth, and effective use of communication technology. However, there are certain dimensions of well-being that are lagging behind due to inequality. For example, rates of unemployment of women are disproportionately high and women's participation in the labor force and political life is still scant. In addition, indicators of freedom of expression, religious tolerance, and happiness are still low in most MENA countries.

The MENA countries have done much to spread and promote public and primary education. Despite the quantitative development of education, in terms of length of time in school and large enrollments of students, in the MENA region, the qualitative dimension of education is lagging.

It is worth mentioning that this study has used multiple (more than 14) indicators and a multidimensional approach to challenge a holistic and overall depiction of quality of life and well-being in the MENA region, particularly when dealing with countries that have different levels of the HDI. For example, out of the selected MENA countries under study in 2015, only two countries, namely Turkey and the Emirates, ranked as having a high HDI value and very high HDI value, respectively, and perform within the expected range on the indicator of "availability of affordable housing" (Social Progress Index 2017). All of the countries made advances in education and health. Some countries, however, need to make other deliberate advances in economic opportunities (employment/jobs) or provisions (housing) to ensure higher rates of well-being and happiness.

Another challenge is that the United Nations Development Programme (2016) and the Social Progress Index (2017) have not addressed well-being indicators and outcomes for different population groups within a country.

This chapter suggests that further studies are needed to assess outcome indicators of quality of life and well-being in the MENA region, especially in light of these politically challenging times to ensure human development process as defined by the United Nations.

References

Central Intelligence Agency. (2015). *The world factbook: United Arab Emirates*. Retrieved from https://www.cia.gov/library/publications/the-world-factbook/geos/print_ae.html.

Central Intelligence Agency. (2018). *The world factbook*. Washington, D.C: Central Intelligence Agency. Retrieved from https://www.cia.gov/library/publications/the-world-factbook/fields/2103.html.

Clifton, J. (2017). The happiest and unhappiest countries in the world. *Gallup World Poll: World Region, Middle East and North Africa*. Retrieved from http://news.gallup.com/opinion/gallup/206468/happiest-unhappiest-countries-world.aspx?g_source=WORLD_REGION_MIDDLE_EAST_NORTH_AFRICA&g_medium=topic&g_campaign=tiles.

Diener, E. (1984). Subjective well-being. *Psychological Bulletin, 95*(3), 542–575.

Drine, I. (2012). 'Successful' development models in the MENA region. United Nations University and World Institute for Development Economics Research, Working Paper No. 2012/52. Retrieved from https://www.wider.unu.edu/publication/'successful'-development-models-mena-region.

Ehsani, K., & Keshavarzian, A. (2018). The moral economy of the Iranian protests. *Jacobin*. Retrieved from: https://www.jacobinmag.com/2018/01/iranian-protests-revolution-rouhani-ahmadinejad.

Eickelman, D. (1992). Mass higher education and the religious imagination in contemporary Arab societies. *American Ethnologist, 19*(4), 643–655.

Eickelman, D. (2008). Gender and religion in the public and private sphere. In K. Ohtsuka & D. F. Eickelman (Eds.), *Crossing boundaries: Gender and the public, and the private in contemporary Muslim societies* (pp. 135–150). Tokyo: Research Institute for Languages and Cultures of Asia and Africa.

Eickelman, D. (2017). Building universities that leads: The Arabian peninsula. In D. Eickelman & R. Abusharaf (Eds.), *Higher education investment in the Arab states of the Gulf: Strategies for excellence and diversity* (pp. 8–22). Berlin: Gerlach Press.

el-Aswad, el-S. (1990). *al-ṣabr fī al-turāth al-sha'ī al-Misrī: dirāsah anthrpolojiyya*, Alexandria: Munsha'at al-Ma'raf.

el-Aswad, el-S. (1993). The Gift and the Image of the Self and the Other Among Rural Egyptians. In Rosa Godula (Ed.), *The Gift in Culture*. (pp 35–49). Krakow: Jagiellonian University Press.
el-Aswad, el-S. (1999). Hierarchy and Symbolic Construction of the Person among Rural Egyptians.*Anthropos*, *94* (4/6), 431–445.
el-Aswad, el-S. (2002). *Religion and folk cosmology: Scenarios of the visible and invisible in rural Egypt*. Westport, CT: Praeger Press.
el-Aswad, el-S. (2004). Viewing the world through Upper Egyptian eyes: From regional crisis to global blessing. In N. Hopkins & R. Saad (Eds.), *Identity and Change in Upper Egypt* (pp. 55–78). Cairo: American University in Cairo Press.
el-Aswad, el-S. (2012). *Muslim worldviews and everyday lives*. Lanham, MD: AltaMira Press, Rowman & Littlefield Publisher.
el-Aswad, el-S. (2014). Communication. In K. Harvey (Ed.), *Encyclopedia of Social Media and Politics* (1: 304–308). Thousand Oaks, CA: Sage.
el-Aswad, el-S. (2016a). Political challenges confronting the Islamic world. In H. Tiliouine & R. J. Estes (Eds.), *The state of social progress of Islamic societies: Social, economic, political, and ideological challenges* (pp. 361–377). Cham, Switzerland: Springer International Publishing. https://doi.org/10.1007/978-3-319-24774-8_16.
el-Aswad, el-S. (2016b). State, nation and Islamism in contemporary Egypt: An anthropological perspective. *Urban Anthropology*, 45(1–2), 63–92.
el-Aswad, el-S. (2016c). Social and spatial organization patterns in the traditional house: A case study of Al Ain City, UAE. In Y. Elsheshtawi (Ed.), *Transformations of the Emirati national house* (pp. 190-203). Abu Dhabi: UAE-Culture Press.
El-Menawy, A. (2017). Egyptians' sense of humor is very telling. *Arab News*. Retrieved from http://www.arabnews.com/node/1165171.
Haybron, D., & Tiberius, V. (2015). Well-being policy: What standard of well-being? *Journal of the American Philosophical Association, 1*(4), 712–733.
Helliwell, J., et al. (2013). *World happiness report 13*. (United Nations). Retrieved from http://worldhappiness.report/wp-content/uploads/sites/2/2013/09/WorldHappinessReport2013_online.pdf.
Helliwell, J., et al. (2016). *World happiness report 2016 update: The distribution of world happiness*. (United Nations). Retrieved from http://worldhappiness.report/wp-content/uploads/sites/2/2016/03/HR-V1Ch2_web.pdf.
Helliwell, J., et al. (2017). *World happiness report 2017: The social foundation of world happiness* (United Nations). Retrieved from http://worldhappiness.report/wp-content/uploads/sites/2/2017/03/HR17-Ch2.pdf.
Huppert, F. A., & Cooper, C. L. (2014). *Interventions and policies to enhance wellbeing: A complete reference guide* (Vol. VI). Chichester, West Sussex: Wiley.
Institute for Health Metrics and Evaluation. (2016a). Egypt. Retrieved from http://www.healthdata.org/egypt.
Institute for Health Metrics and Evaluation. (2016b). Iran. Retrieved from http://www.healthdata.org/iran.
Institute for Health Metrics and Evaluation. (2016c). Israel. Retrieved from http://www.healthdata.org/israel.
Institute for Health Metrics and Evaluation. (2016d). Tunisia. Retrieved from http://www.healthdata.org/tunisia.
Institute for Health Metrics and Evaluation. (2016e). Turkey. Retrieved from http://www.healthdata.org/turkey.
Institute for Health Metrics and Evaluation. (2016f). United Arab Emirates. Retrieved from http://www.healthdata.org/united-arab-emirates.
International Labor Organization. (2017). Tunisia. Retrieved from http://www.ilo.org/dyn/normlex/en/f?p=NORMLEXPUB:11110:0::NO::P11110_COUNTRY_ID:102986.
Keyes, C. L. (1998). Social well-being. *Social Psychology Quarterly, 61*(2), 121–140.
Lin, E. (2016). The subjective list theories. *Australasian Journal of Philosophy, 94*(1), 99–114.

McGillivray, M., & Clarke, M. (2007). Human well-being: Concepts and measures. In M. McGillivray & M. Clarke (Eds.), *Understanding human well-being* (pp. 3–16). Tokyo, New York, Paris: United Nations University Press.

Organization for Economic Cooperation and Development. (2013). *OECD guidelines on measuring subjective well-being*. Paris: OECD Publishing. https://doi.org/10.1787/9789264191655-en.

Organization for Economic Co-operation and Development. (2015). *Measuring and assessing well-being in Israel.* Paris: OECD Publishing. doi.org/https://doi.org/10.1787/9789264246034-en. Retrieved from http://mof.gov.il/chiefecon/internationalconnections/oecd/oecd_wellbeingreport.pdf.

Silva, J., Levin, V., & Morgand, M. (2012). *The way forward for social safety nets in the Middle East and North Africa*. Washington D.C: World Bank.

Sirgy, M. J. (2011). Theoretical perspectives guiding QOL indicator projects. *Social Indicators Research, 103,* 1–22.

Sirgy, M. J., Estes, R. J., & Selian, A. N. (2017). How we measure well-being: The data behind the history of well-being. In R. J. Estes & M. J. Sirgy (Eds.), *The pursuit of human well-being: The untold global history* (pp. 135–160). Dordrecht, NL: Springer.

Smith-Spark, L. (2018). Tunisia protests: Why are people taking to the streets? Retrieved from CNN: http://www.cnn.com/2018/01/10/africa/tunisia-protests-intl/index.html.

Social Progress Index. (2016). *Social progress imperatives: Executive summary.* Retrieved from http://www.socialprogressimperative.org/wp-content/uploads/2016/06/SPI-2016-Main-Report.pdf.

Social Progress Index. (2017). *Social progress imperatives*. Retrieved from http://www.socialprogressindex.com/assets/downloads/resources/en/English-2017-Social-Progress-Index-Findings-Report_embargo-d-until-June-21-2017.pdf.

UNESCO. (2015). *Education for All 2015 National Review Report: Egypt*. Retrieved from http://unesdoc.unesco.org/images/0022/002299/229905e.pdf.

UNESCO. (2016). Institute for Statistics. Retrieved from http://uis.unesco.org/en/country/EG.

UNESCO. (2018a). Egypt. Retrieved from http://uis.unesco.org/en/country/EG.

UNESCO. (2018b). Iran. Retrieved from http://uis.unesco.org/en/country/ir.

UNESCO. (2018c). Israel. Retrieved from http://uis.unesco.org/en/country/il.

UNESCO. (2018d). Tunisia. Retrieved from http://uis.unesco.org/en/country/tn.

UNESCO. (2018e). Turkey. Retrieved from http://uis.unesco.org/en/country/tr.

UNESCO. (2018f). United Arab Emirates. Retrieved from http://uis.unesco.org/en/country/ae.

United Arab Emirates. (2017). (Cabinet). Retrieved from https://uaecabinet.ae/en/details/cabinet-members/her-excellency-ohoud-bint-khalfan-al-roumi.

UNICEF. (2006). The state of the world's children 2007: Women and children: the double dividend of gender equality. Retrieved from https://books.google.com/books?hl=en&lr=&id=HiIZr4QFkOMC&oi=fnd&pg=PR6&dq=UNICEF+HIV+prevalence+in+Iran+2000+&ots=16J-Lj2Q8l&sig=qwqlNw_P4IyPSg1ai1lggarl8_8#v=onepage&q=UNICEF%20HIV%20prevalence%20in%20Iran%202000&f=false.

UNICEF. (2013). Israel. Retrieved from https://www.unicef.org/infobycountry/israel_statistics.html.

UNICEF. (2015). Egypt. Retrieved from https://www.unicef.org/egypt/hiv_aids.html.

United Nations. (2018). *The Sustainable Development Goals 2015–2030.* United Nations Association of Philadelphia. Retrieved from http://una-gp.org/the-sustainable-development-goals-2015-2030/.

United Nations Development Programme. (2002). *Human development report 2002: Deepening democracy in a fragmented world*. Retrieved from http://hdr.undp.org/sites/default/files/reports/263/hdr_2002_en_complete.pdf

United Nations Development Programme. (2016a). *Human Development Index*. Retrieved from http://hdr.undp.org/en/indicators/137506.

United Nations Development Programme. (2016b) *Human Development Report 2016: Human development for everyone*. Retrieved from http://hdr.undp.org/sites/default/files/HDR2016_EN_Overview_Web.pdf.
Veenhoven, R. (2017). Average happiness in 158 nations 2005–2014. *World Database of Happiness. Rank report average happiness*. Retrieved from http://worlddatabaseofhappiness.eur.nl/hap_nat/findingreports/RankReport_AverageHappiness.php.
World Bank. (2017). *General government final consumption expenditure (% of GDP)*. Retrieved from https://data.worldbank.org/indicator/NE.CON.GOVT.ZS.
World Bank. (2018a). Iran. Retrieved from http://www.worldbank.org/en/country/iran/overview.
World Bank. (2018b). *Israel: Poverty headcount ratio at $1.90 a day (2011 PPP) (% of population)* Retrieved from https://data.worldbank.org/indicator/SI.POV.DDAY?locations=IL.
World Bank. (2018c). *Turkey. Poverty headcount ratio at $1.90 a day (2011 PPP) (% of population)*. Retrieved from https://data.worldbank.org/indicator/SI.POV.DDAY?locations=TR.
World Health Organization. (2016a). Egypt: *Maternal mortality in 1990–2015. Egypt*. Retrieved from http://www.who.int/gho/maternal_health/countries/egy.pdf.
World Health Organization. (2016b). *Iran: Maternal mortality in 1990–2015*. Retrieved from http://www.who.int/gho/maternal_health/countries/irn.pdf.
World Health Organization.(2016c). *Israel: Maternal mortality in 1990–2015*. Retrieved from http://www.who.int/gho/maternal_health/countries/isr.pdf.
World Health Organization. (2016d). *Tunisia: Maternal mortality in 1990–2015*. Retrieved from http://www.who.int/gho/maternal_health/countries/tun.pdf.
World Health Organization. (2016e). Turkey: *Maternal mortality in 1990–2015*. Retrieved from http://www.who.int/gho/maternal_health/countries/tur.pdf.
World Health Organization. (2016f). United Arab Emirates: *Maternal mortality in 1990–2015*. Retrieved from http://www.who.int/gho/maternal_health/countries/are.pdf.
World Health Organization. (2017). *World Health Statistics 2017: Monitoring health for the SDGS, Sustainable Development Goals*. Retrieved from http://apps.who.int/iris/bitstream/10665/255336/1/9789241565486-eng.pdf?ua=1.
World Health Organization. (2018). *Global health observatory (GHO) data: Life expectancy*. Retrieved from http://www.who.int/gho/mortality_burden_disease/life_tables/situation_trends_text/en/.

Chapter 5
Key Drivers of Well-Being and Policy Issues in the Middle East and North Africa Region

Abstract This chapter investigates the staging of the drivers of well-being and social-public policies in the region of the Middle East and North Africa (MENA). This study provides an assessment of the roles of economic and non-economic drivers related to health, education, economy, and technology in shaping policy priorities and the policy options available to the MENA region. The objective of this inquiry is to show to what extent the drivers and input indicators of well-being help the governments and policy makers generate sociocultural plans and public policies aimed at improving the quality of life the people living in the MENA region. This study proposes that a better understanding of the drivers and determinants of well-being in the MENA region will provide relevant considerations concerning policy issues.

Keywords Well-being · Drivers · Policy issues · Human development MENA region

5.1 Introduction

The previous chapters, particularly Chap. 4, have addressed the outcome indicators showing progress in quality of life and well-being in the selected Middle East and North Africa (MENA) countries represented in the increase in the expected years at birth, adult literacy, expected years of schooling, mean years of schooling, and gross domestic product (GDP) per capita. The goal of this chapter is to provide data analyses concerning the drivers or input indicators that impact the quality of life and well-being in the MENA countries at the national and regional levels. It also seeks to use these input indicators of quality of life to assess progress in the domains of health, education, economy, and technology, among others. In brief, key drivers or input indicators help explain the improvement in the Human Development Index values of the selected MENA countries discussed in Chap. 4.

Well-being can be viewed as an overarching policy initiative that combines economic and non-economic goals into a single framework for the benefit of people

el-S. el-Aswad, *The Quality of Life and Policy Issues among the Middle East and North African Countries*, Human Well-Being Research and Policy Making,
https://doi.org/10.1007/978-3-030-00326-5_5

(Keyes 1998; Lammy and Tyler 2014). The drive to improve peoples' quality of life is global. For decades, policy makers, political leaders, educators, medical professionals, and businessmen worldwide have focused on issues of how to advance the well-being of their citizens. A better understanding of the drivers and determinants of well-being in the MENA region will provide relevant recommendations concerning policy issues. In other words, well-being drivers and information provide policy makers and development scholars with a useful way for addressing policy priorities. Well-being research has significant policy implications. And, adequate social-public policy plays a critical role in improving peoples' well-being and quality of life.

Social policy refers to plans or programs designed by the political system and the private sector to both solve public problems confronting the society and achieve the objectives pursued by the greater population. Social policy is a deeply political process of sociocultural production engaged in and shaped by social actors in different locations who exert remarkable amounts of influence. These actors differ in their authority to define what is problematic in well-being, shape the explanations and means of how problems should be resolved, and determine how the image of future change efforts should be directed (Hamann and Rosen 2011).

5.2 Brief History

Middle Eastern states have implemented an array of policies since the 1940s and 1950s, driven by the primacy of nation-building and state legitimization. The major redistribution policies during these periods of time have included the nationalization of foreign assets and domestic enterprises, land reform, mass education, and the support of low-income groups through direct financial transfers by the state. During the 1960s and 1980s MENA countries benefited from high rates of public spending, planning, and implementation of social-public policies including free education, health insurance, retirement compensation, maternity pay, free hospital care, and consumer subsidies, particularly for basic food items and housing (Jawad 2008; Karshenas and Moghadam 2009). Since the 1990s, due to economic problems and the diminishing role of the state as a provider of jobs and supplier of social services, the majority of MENA states have made structural adjustment programs that have negatively affected the poor. However, social-public policies have witnessed some improvement since 2000 in that about 30–40% of the population has been covered by formal social security plans. Less than that was covered by NGOs or private agencies of social welfare (Jawad 2015).

As a part of social policy, public spending by governments in the MENA region has played an important role in social development. Higher public spending on social welfare is associated with higher well-being at the national level (Huppert and Cooper 2014). Social policies have become the vehicle for implementing redistributive programs in MENA states (Yousef 2004). Furthermore, spending on social safety nets in the MENA region as a whole have increased from 10.1% of the total expenditure before the global economic crisis of 2009, to 11.9% during the crisis, and then to 12.5% afterwards, which reflects 4.16%, 4.44%, and 4.59% of the GDP, respectively (Jawad 2015).

As the outcomes of well-being are different in the MENA countries, public-social policies are also different. The pathway to achieve well-being outcomes involves recognizing the importance of social drivers that are related not only to poverty reduction (Sachs 2005) but also to enhanced capacity for productivity and employment, social justice, and the empowerment of disadvantaged groups, women, smallholders, and informal economy workers (United Nations Research Institute for Social Development 2013).

5.3 Key Drivers

The data of key drivers of well-being and policy issues presented in the following sections have a double objective. On the one hand, they deal with factors yielding positive aspects or outcomes of quality of life that policy makers seek to maintain and increase. On the other, some data tackle shortcomings or negative elements hindering the realization of well-being that policy makers strive to eliminate or decrease. Using well-being input "data can improve the quality of evidence on which policy is based, helping policymakers to better predict the impact of policy on people's lives" (Lammy and Tyler 2014: 3).

As is shown in the subsequent sections, the drivers of well-being and policy issues in the MENA region vary according to the types of government and non-government agencies and actors in each country.

5.3.1 Key Drivers in Egypt

I discuss in this section key drivers of well-being in relation to health, education, economic well-being, communication technology, religious tolerance, and political right in Egypt.

5.3.1.1 Health Well-Being in Egypt

Regionally, most MENA countries have universal public health care systems designed and financed by general government revenues. Life expectancy at birth, discussed in Chap. 3, has increased in the MENA region due to the improvement of medical technology and health care expenditures. In 2014, health spending per capita in the MENA region was about $870 (5.2% per GDP) (Financing Global Health 2016). And the region is expected to display "the fastest health care spending growth globally, at around 9.3% annually in 2015–2019" (Deloitte 2016).

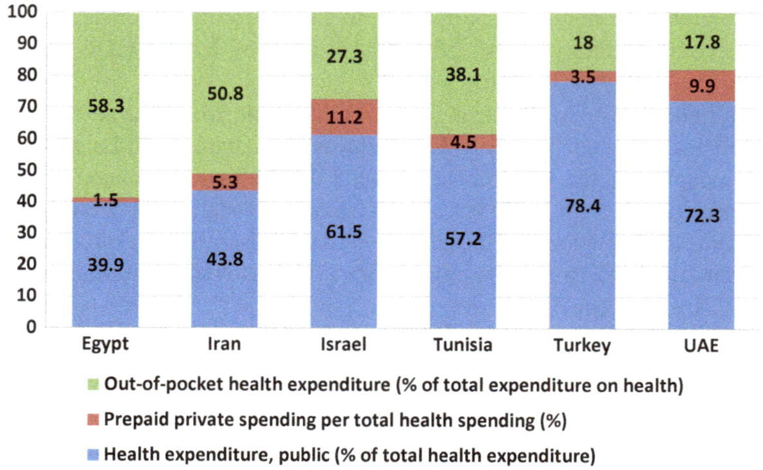

Fig. 5.1 Health spending by source in the Middle East and North Africa Region, 2014–2015 (Data from Financing Global Health 2016; World Bank 2018a)

Egypt has spared no effort to build and finance health care systems as fundamental drivers impacting the quality of life and well-being of Egyptian citizens. The Ministry of Health and Population (MOHP) is responsible for overall health and population policy as well as for the provision of primary, preventive, and curative care. The MOHP oversees and manages more than 5000 health facilities and 80,000 beds nationwide (World Health Organization 2018). Other organizations such as the Health Insurance Organization, the Curative Care Organization, and the Teaching Hospitals and Institutes Organization constitute quasi-governmental sectors collaborating with the MOHP. Private sectors form the third component of the health system in Egypt (Ministry of Health and Population, Egypt 2018).

In 2015, the health spending per capita (purchasing power parity [PPP]) in Egypt was around $581 (Table 5.1 and Fig. 5.1). The total health expenditure (public and private) reached 5.6% of the total GDP. The public health expenditure in 2014 reached 2.2% of the total GDP (compared to 1.8% in 1990) (United Nations Development Programme 2016a; World Health Organization 2017). The government health spending was about 39.9% of total health expenditure, while out-of-pocket spending reached 58.3% of total health spending (highest among the selected MENA countries). Prepaid private spending comprised 1.5% of total health spending. The annualized rate of change in total health spending per capita for 1995–2014 was 5.5% (Financing Global Health 2016; World Data Atlas 2018a) (Fig. 5.2).

Although the expenditure on health is not as good as it could be, there are serious attempts to improve the health well-being in Egyptian society. In other words, over the past three decades, Egypt has made significant progress in developing its public health infrastructure and medical services, particularly in the areas of prenatal care, child immunization, diseases, water, and sanitation. The government of Egypt is

Table 5.1 Health spending by source in the Middle East and North Africa region, 2014–2015 (Data from World Bank 2018a and Financing Global Health 2016)

Country	Total health spending per capita (2015 purchasing power parity dollars)	Total health expenditure (% of GDP) public and private	Public-government health expenditure (% of GDP)	Health expenditure, public (% of total health expenditure)	Prepaid private spending per total health spending (%)	Out-of-pocket health expenditure (% of total expenditure on health)	Annualized rate of change in total health spending per capita, 1995–2014 (%)
Egypt	$581.0	5.6	2.2	39.9	1.5	58.3	5.5
Iran	$1073.0	6.9	2.8	43.8	5.3	50.8	6.2
Israel	$2722.0	7.7	4.8	61.5	11.2	27.3	1.9
Tunisia	$791.0	7.0	4.0	57.2	4.5	38.1	3.5
Turkey	$1040.0	5.4	4.2	78.4	3.5	18.0	6.6
UAE	$2561.0	3.6	2.6	72.3	9.9	17.8	0.4

GDP gross domestic product

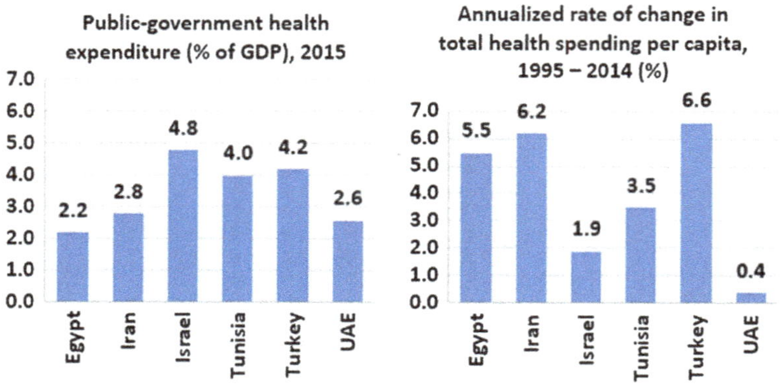

Fig. 5.2 Public-government health expenditure (% of GDP) and annualized rate change in selected MENA countries (Data extracted from World bank 2018a; Financing Global Health 2016)

reforming social health insurance and improving health care financing particularly for the poor and those living in underprivileged areas (United Nations Development Assistance Framework 2013).

Egyptian women receive prenatal services provided by physicians and skilled medical professionals. For instance, prenatal care reached 90.30% in 2014 (compared to 52.10% in 1991), which was higher than the worldwide rate of 83.85% recorded in the same year (UNICEF 2017; World Bank 2018a). The mandatory paid maternity leave was 90 days, sustaining the mother and child after delivery. The rate of fully immunized children (receiving the bacillus Calmette–Guérin [BCG] vaccine against tuberculosis, the measles vaccine, or the measles-mumps-rubella (MMR) vaccine, three vaccinations against diphtheria, pertussis, and tetanus (DPT), and three doses of polio vaccine) reached 91.0% in 2014 (UNICEF 2016a). In 2015, the percentage of infants (percentage of 1-year-olds) lacking DTP immunization was reduced to 4.0%, whereas the rate of infants lacking measles immunization dropped to 7.0% (United Nations Development Programme 2016a) (Table 5.2).

Another example showcasing the development in medical services has been the establishment of the National Committee for Control of Viral Hepatitis to instigate an integrated nationwide policy to provide patient care and ensure global access to the hepatitis C virus, an infectious and life-threatening disease causing a tremendous economic burden in Egypt in 2015, estimated at US $3.81 billion (Gomaa et al. 2017).

Table 5.2 shows that physician density in Egypt has fluctuated through the years. For example, there were 2.83 physicians per 1000 people in 2010 compared to 1.84 physicians per 1000 people in 1994 (World Bank 2018d). However, it reached 0.81 physicians per 1000 people in 2014 (Central Intelligence Agency 2018), lower than the worldwide rate of 1.85 physicians per 1000 (World Bank 2018d). It is to be noted that the World Health Organization (2017) estimated that at least 2.5 physicians per 1000 people are needed to provide adequate coverage with primary care interventions

Table 5.2 Drivers of health in the Middle East and North Africa Region (Data from the Central Intelligence Agency 2018; UNDP 2016a; World Bank 2018a, b, c, d; World Health Organization 2016, 2017)

Country	Physician density (per 1000 people)	Prenatal care (%)	Maternity leave (days)	Immunization (% 1-year-olds)	Safe drinking water (% 1000 of population)	Improved sanitation (% 1000 of population)
Egypt	1.84 (1994) 2.83 (2010) 0.81 (2014)	52.10 (1991) 90.30 (2014)	90 (2015)	91.0 (2014)	99.4 (2015)	94.7(2015)
Iran	0.88 (2005) 0.89 (2010) 1.49 (2014)	91.50 (2000) 96.90 (2010)	270 (2015)	94.0 (2014)	96.2% (2015)	90 (2011)
Israel	3.76 (2000) 3.44 (2010) 3.57 (2015)	NA	98 (2015)	94.6 (2014)	100 (2015)	100 (2015)
Tunisia	0.54 (1990) 0.67 (2000) 1.29 (2015)	91.5 (2000) 98.1 (2012)	30 (2015)	93.0 (2014)	97 (2014)	94 (2014)
Turkey	0.94 (1990) 1.44 (2000) 1.75 (2014)	62.2 (1993) 96.9 (2013)	112 (2015)	94.4 (2014)	100 (2015)	98.3 (2015)
UAE	1.56 (2015)	98.9 (2004) 100 (2015)	45 (2015)	95.0 (2014)	99.6 (2015)	98 (2015)

(Fig. 5.3). Despite this limitation, Egyptians have good access to key public utilities. Safe drinking water is 99.4% available in Egypt (100% in urban environment and 99% in rural areas) (Fig. 5.4). Similarly, 94.7% of the population (96.8% in urban and 93.1% in rural communities) has had access to improved and safe sanitation facilities since 2015 (World Health Organization 2017).

The health care system is supported by further future policies aimed at improving the health well-being of the Egyptian people. According to Egypt's "2030 Vision" for sustainable development (El-Megharbel 2015, 15), the government is planning to achieve equitable access to 80% of essential health interventions by 2030 as well as to extend medical insurance to farmers and agriculture workers who do not have access to public health insurance programs. Although notable progress has been made in basic public health provisions, further expansion will require greater investment from both the state and private industry. The government needs to meet its commitments to increase public spending on health initiatives in order to make progress on the goals for quality and equitable health care access.

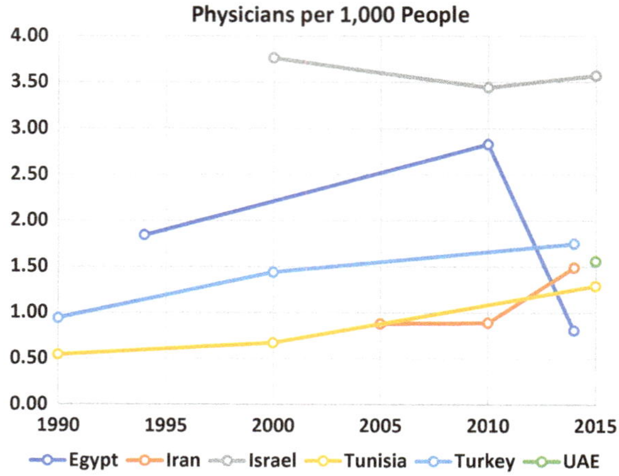

Fig. 5.3 Physician density in selected MENA countries, 1990–2015 (Data extracted from Financing Global Health 2016; World Bank 2018a)

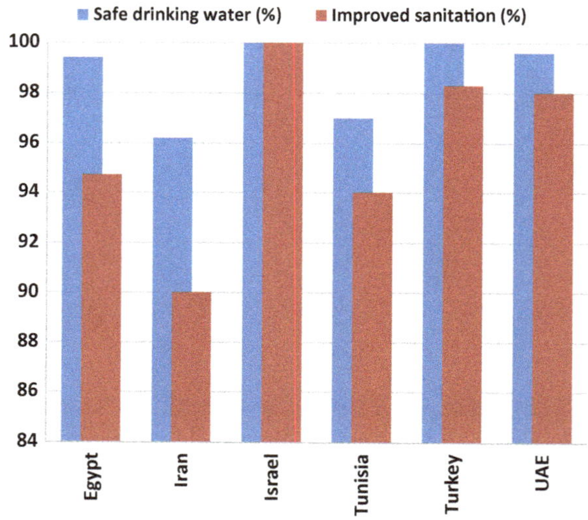

Fig. 5.4 Drinking water and sanitation in the selected Middle East and North Africa countries, 1990–2015 (Data from Financing Global Health 2016; World Bank 2018a)

5.3.1.2 Educational Well-Being in Egypt

Around the world, there are strong links between education, better health outcomes, and longer lives. In Egypt, as in other countries, education is an essential driver of overall well-being. Education promotes healthier lives and enables people to exercise influence beyond the nation's borders through participating in the global economy and impacting decisions taken on a global measure (World Bank 2018b).

Egypt's public education system is the largest in the MENA region in terms of the magnitude of the student populations. There are around 51,000 public schools, 9000 Al-Azhar schools, and 8000 private schools in Egypt, including more than 100 internationally affiliated schools (Oxford Business Group 2018). Compulsory education lasts 12 years and extends from age 6 to age 17. In Egypt, children have more access to quality basic education (formal and non-formal), with a special focus on vulnerable groups and gender equality (United Nations Development Assistance Framework 2013).

Table 5.3 shows that public expenditure on education was about 3.8% of the GDP in 2008 to 2012. The following data highlight how in some ways Egypt structured its financial and educational resources to address educational well-being. By 2015, the average annual spending per pupil was around $300 (UNESCO 2018a) (Fig. 5.5). By 2014–2015, class density for primary school reached 44.2 students per classroom, whereas that for secondary school was 39.3 students per classroom. The pupil-teacher ratio in primary schools in 2014 was 23 pupils per teacher and primary school teachers trained to teach was at 73%. The primary school dropout rate was about 0.6%, whereas the preparatory school dropout rate reached 4.5% in 2013–2014 (UNICEF 2016a; United Nations Development Programme 2016a) (Fig. 5.6).

Improving educational outcomes requires understanding the impact of educational policies as well as that of other policies (e.g., social and political) and non-policy drivers (e.g., socioeconomic environment and cultural background, for instance) on pupils' learning (Organization for Economic Cooperation and Development 2015a, b). In April 2018, the World Bank announced a 5-year initiative of US $500 million, aligned with Egypt's "2030 Vision," to support Egypt's education reform. The initiative aims to expand access to quality kindergarten education for around 500,000 children, train 500,000 teachers and education officials, and provide 1.5 million students and teachers with digital learning resources (World Bank 2018c).

Egypt is known for having a young generation where those below 14 years old make up 33.29% of the population, and the proportion of 15- to 24-year-olds comprise 18.94% of the population. This statement implies that ensuring access to education for these large youth cohorts will secure well-being outcomes in the future. The Ministry of Education appointed 30,000 new teachers in March 2015 to teach and train students enrolled in 1150 new schools (Oxford Business Group 2018). However, Egypt achieved a score of 2.6 (7 = high) and was globally ranked 113 (out of 138 countries) on the indicator of "Internet access in schools" (Fig. 5.7). Meanwhile, Egypt ranked 134 and 112 on the indicators of the "quality of primary education" and "quality of the higher education," respectively, in the 2015–2016 *Global Competitiveness Index* (World Economic Forum 2017: 168).

The present government has focused on reforming the education system through updating curricula, training teachers, reducing classroom sizes, building new classrooms, reducing the number of student dropouts, developing technological skills of both instructors and students, and improving school facilities. It is expected that Egypt will in time achieve universal primary education for both genders and will successfully reduce the illiteracy rate (Oxford Business Group 2018).

Teachers are key actors in education, and policy makers need to pay more attention to improving quality of instruction and increasing destitute wages, particularly in places with meager economic resources such as Egypt so that external sources of income do not need to be sought. The government should offer free lessons as a short-term solution to the need for private tuition (tutoring), develop a child friendly curriculum, and increase varied school activities. The government should also link

Table 5.3 Drivers of education and global rank in the Middle East and North Africa Region (Data from the UNDP 2016a; UNESCO 2018a, b; World Economic Forum 2017)

Country	Public expenditure (% of GDP)	Average cost per primary student (US$)	Classroom size (students per classroom)	Pupil-teacher ratio (primary school)	Internet access in schools		Quality of primary education (2015–2016)		Quality of higher education (2015–2016)	
					Score (1 = low; 7 = high)	Rank 138 countries	Score (1 = low; 7 = high)	Rank 138 countries	Score (1 = low; 7 = high)	Rank 138 countries
Egypt	3.8 (2012)	300 (2015)	39 (2015)	23 (2015)	2.6	133	2.1	134	2.6	112
Iran	2.8 (2015) 3.76 (2016)	1363 (2015)	NA	26 (2015)	3.5	113	4.1	65	3.3	97
Israel	6.19 (2000) 5.74 (2014)	7273 (2014)	27 (2015)	13 (2015)	5.3	27	4.5	45	4.7	24
Tunisia	6.6 (2015)	1674 (2015)	31 (2015)	17 (2015)	3.5	112	3.6	85	3.1	107
Turkey	4.77 (2014)	3316 (2014)	23 (2015)	20 (2015)	4.1	79	3.1	105	3.2	104
UAE	1.22 (1997) NA (2015)	NA	NA	19 (2015)	6.1	4	5.5	12	5.3	10

GDP gross domestic product

databases of enrolled students at the Ministry of Education and Al-Azhar Education as well as the civil registry databases to identify out-of-school children (UNICEF-OOSCI 2018).

5.3.1.3 Economic Well-Being in Egypt

Due to the political and social unrest following the 2011 revolution, Egypt's economy has suffered considerably as a result of the drastic impact on the tourism sector, a decrease in foreign investments, and shrinkage of foreign reserves. However, the economy is gradually improving, and the annual rates of GDP growth have improved from an average of 2% during the period 2010/11–2013/14 to an average of 4.3% in 2015/2016, driven by investments, exports, and consumption (World Bank 2017a).

Despite its economic problems, Egypt extended eligibility criteria for subsidized food supplies and cash transfers to vulnerable populations, which led to greater access to foodstuffs and monetary resources (Arab Barometer 2011, 2013; Bremer 2015; Jawad 2015). Egypt's general government final consumption expenditure in 2015 was 11.8% of the total GDP. Despite the regression in the agricultural activities, employment in agriculture was 28.0% of the total employment in 2015. Meanwhile, the overall employment-to-population ratio in 2015 was 43.5% (ages 15 and older). The labor force participation rate (ages 15 and older) was 49.4%. Child labor (ages 5–14) is still high in Egypt, reaching 7.0% (United Nations Development Programme 2016b). In Egypt as in other Muslim societies, family obligations and loyalty to one's parents and kin play an important role in sustaining an informal economy that, in turn, supports the needy (Eickelman and Piscatori 1996).

The role of nation-state governments is to look for effective means to generate economic resources to promote people's quality of life and well-being. The Egyptian

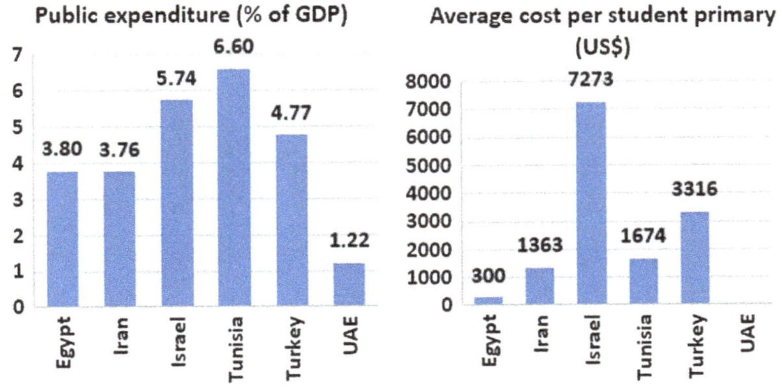

Fig. 5.5 Public expenditure (percent of gross domestic product) and average cost per student primary (US$) in selected Middle East and North Africa countries (Data from Financing Global Health 2016; World Bank 2018a)

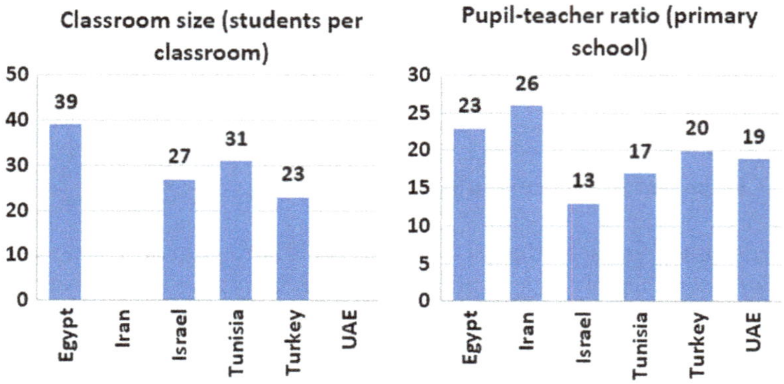

Fig. 5.6 Classroom size and pupil-teacher ratio in selected Middle East and North Africa countries (Data from Organization for Economic Cooperation and Development 2015a, b; UNESCO 2018a, b; UNICEF 2016a, b)

government implemented a transformational reforms program, reducing energy subsidies, liberating the Egyptian pound, and attracting local and foreign investments among other economic initiatives. According to the *Global Competitiveness Report* of 2015–2016, the market size in Egypt was globally ranked 25 (out of 138 countries), a larger market than that of neighboring countries (World Economic Forum 2017). However, Egypt fell within the lower half of the global rankings on the indicators of "institutions" (87) and "infrastructure" (96); it especially needs to improve in the domains of macroeconomic environment (134) and innovation (122) (Fig. 5.8).

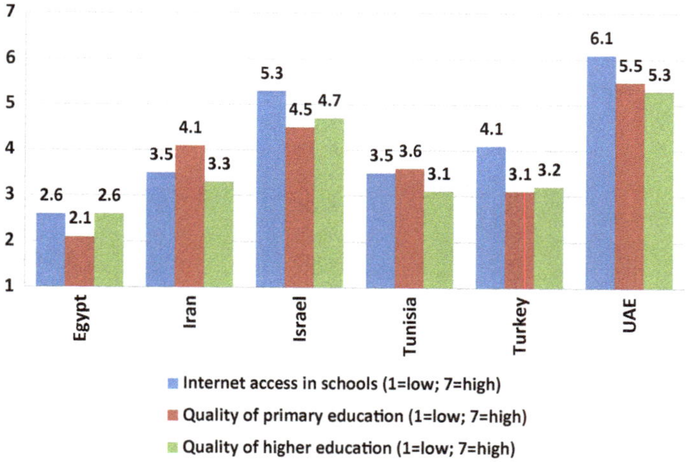

Fig. 5.7 Internet access and quality of education in selected Middle East and North Africa countries (Data from Internet Live Stats 2016)

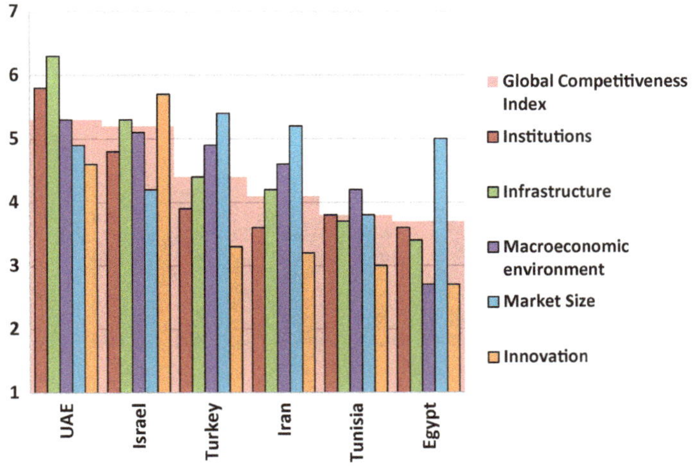

Fig. 5.8 Global Competitiveness Index, ranking of six Middle East and North Africa countries 2016–2017 UAE = United Arab Emirates (Data from World Economic Forum 2017)

Egypt is the most populous MENA country, and its fast-growing population negatively affects its economy and debilitates the distribution of wealth among people. Although Egypt was ranked in the upper half of the global competitiveness rankings (63 out of 138 countries and second out of the six MENA countries) on of the indicator of "burden of government regulation," the state performance including policy making, methods of spending, government debt, and bureaucracy forms one of the essential drivers that negatively impact the overall well-being in the country (World Economic Forum 2017) (Figs. 5.9 and 5.10).

5.3.1.4 Communication Technology in Egypt

Technology indicators refer to the contribution of technological innovations, particularly information technology to quality of life, societal progress, and well-being in a society at large (Sirgy et al. 2017). Communication technology has had a large impact in terms of the current well-being of people in Egypt. According to the *Networked Readiness Index* 2015, measuring the propensity for countries to utilize the opportunities offered by information and communications technology (ICT), Egypt was globally ranked 96 (out of 139 countries) and 6 among the selected MENA countries. However, for the domain of "ICT use and government efficiency," Egypt was globally ranked 112. Concerning the domain of the "availability of latest technologies," Egypt underperformed with a rank of 120 worldwide and 6 among the selected MENA countries (World Economic Forum 2016: 90) (Table 5.4).

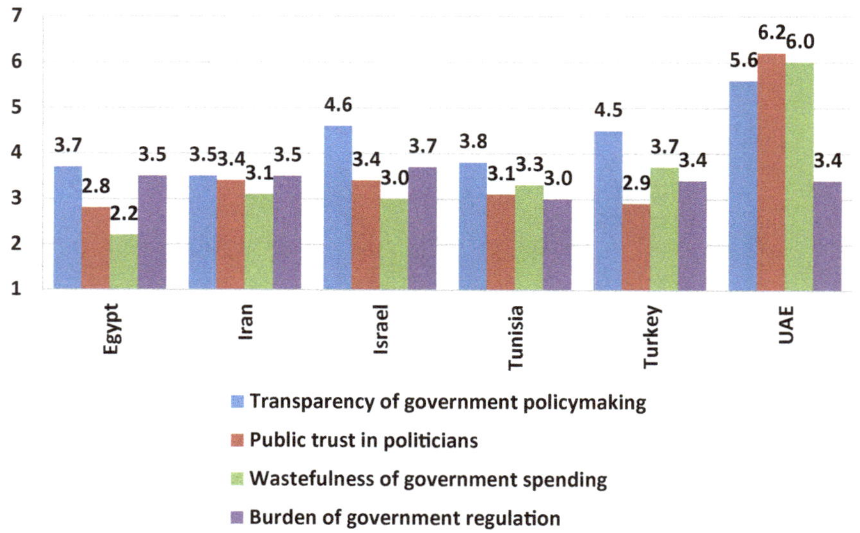

Fig. 5.9 Selected indicators of policy making and governance in the Middle East and North Africa region, 2015–2016 UAE = United Arab Emirates (Data from World Economic Forum 2017)

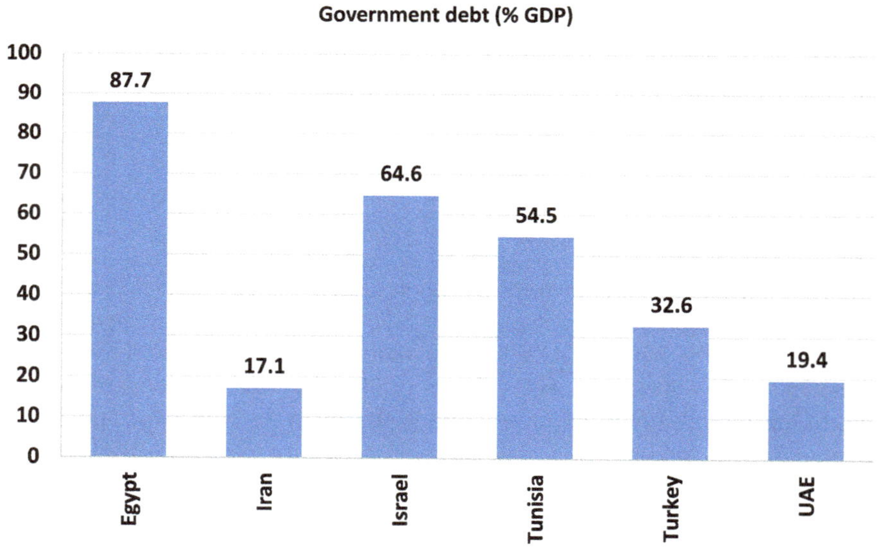

Fig. 5.10 Indicator of government debt in the Middle East and North Africa region, 2015–2016 UAE = United Arab Emirates (Data from World Economic Forum 2017)

5.3.1.5 Religious Tolerance and Political/Human Rights in Egypt

According to the *Social Progress Index* (2017), Egypt performed on the indicator of religious tolerance with a grade of 2 out of 4, but it underperformed on the indicator of freedom of religion with a score of 1 out of 4 (1 = low; 4 = high). Egypt also underperformed on the indicator of political rights with a score of 9 out of 40 (40 = full rights) (Fig. 5.11). On the indicator of political terror, Egypt did not perform well, attaining a rate of 4 out of 5 (5 = high); on the indicator of the level of violent crime, Egypt scored 3.5 out of 5 (5 = high). Furthermore, Egypt scored very low or 5 out of 16 (16 = full freedom) on the indicator of freedom of expression. However, Egypt performed within the lower half of the rankings on the indicator of corruption scoring 34 out of 100 (100 = low) (Table 5.5 and Fig. 5.12).

Table 5.4 Networked readiness index of information and communications technology in the Middle East and North Africa Region (Global Rank out of 139 Countries), 2015 (Data extracted from the Global Information Technology Report 2016 [World Economic Forum 2016])

Rank	Country	Importance of ICT to gov't vision	Gov't success in ICT promotion	Impact of ICTs on access to basic services	Availability of latest technologies	ICT use and gov't efficiency
21	Israel	26	22	21	8	32
26	UAE	1	1	4	9	1
48	Turkey	73	73	46	83	43
81	Tunisia	90	83	110	55	92
92	Iran	91	90	91	111	63
96	Egypt	112	99	108	120	112

ICT information and communications technology; *gov't* government; *UAE* United Arab Emirates

Table 5.5 Human rights and religious tolerance in selected Middle East and North Africa Countries (Data from Social Progress Index 2017)

Country	Religious tolerance (1 = low; 4 = high)	Freedom of religion (1 = low; 4 = high)	Freedom of expression (0 = no freedom; 16 = full freedom)	Political rights (0 = no rights; 40 = full rights)	Political terror (1 = low; 5 = high)	Level of violent crime (1 = low; 5 = high)	Corruption (0 = high; 100 = low)
Egypt	2	1	5	9	4	3.5	34
Iran	2	1	2	7	3.5	2	29
Israel	1	2	12	36	2	2	64
Tunisia	2	2	13	36	2	2	41
Turkey	2	1	6	18	3.5	3	41
UAE	3	3	4	7	2.5	1	66

UAE United Arab Emirates

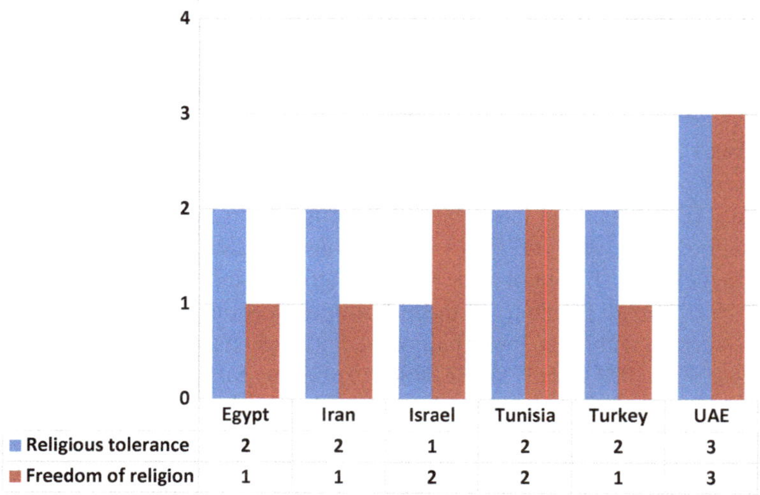

Fig. 5.11 Religious tolerance and freedom of religion in selected Middle East and North Africa countries UAE = United Arab Emirates (Data from Social Progress Index 2017)

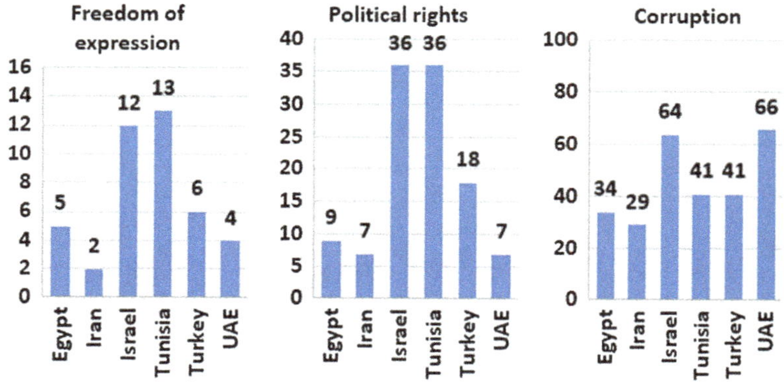

Fig. 5.12 Freedom of expression, political rights, and corruption in selected Middle East and North Africa countries UAE = United Arab Emirates (Data from Social Progress Index 2017)

Egypt needs to maximize its policy issues and reform efforts addressing corruption and major government rigidities that plague the well-being of the majority of people. Overall, social-public policies should be revised to make clear that promoting people's well-being is the overarching objective of the government's planning system.

5.3.2 *Key Drivers in Iran*

I discuss in this section key drivers of well-being in relation to health, education, economic well-being, communication technology, religious tolerance, and political right in Iran.

5.3.2.1 Health Well-Being in Iran

The Ministry of Health and Medical Education (MOHME) is responsible for oversight of the health system in Iran. Other providers of health care include private and non-governmental organizations. Medical schools are under the supervision of the MOHME. Setting health services fees, strictly regulated by the government, is, however, the responsibility of the Supreme Insurance Council, which consists of representatives from the MOHME, insurance corporations, and other economic and governmental bodies (World Bank 2008).

Iran has made major improvements in health care due to the implementation and increase of multiple health drivers related to and including health expenditure, prenatal care, child immunization, fighting communicable and non-communicable diseases, sanitation, and safe water among other medical services. For instance, per capita health spending reached $1073 in 2015, more than double of that of Egypt. Table 5.1 shows that the total health expenditure (public and private) in Iran was 6.9% of the GDP in 2014 whereas the public or government health spending reached 2.8% of the GDP. The government health spending was 43.8% of total health spending, while out of pocket spending reached 50.8% of total health spending (Financing Global Health 2016). It is worth noting that out-of-pocket spending on health in Egypt (58.3%), Iran (50.8%), and Tunisia (38.1%) is higher than that in the other selected MENA countries (Table 5.1). Iran's social health insurance as a share of current health expenditure was at a level of 26.9% in 2015, up from 25.4% from the previous year (World Data Atlas 2018b) (Figs. 5.1 and 5.2).

Table 5.2 shows that the percentage of pregnant women receiving prenatal care in Iran increased from 91.5% in 2000 to 96.90% in 2010 (World Bank 2018a). However, the mandatory paid maternity leave in 2015 was 270 days, higher than that of other MENA countries (United Nations Development Programme 2016a). Furthermore, prenatal health care, counseling nutritional support, and health education play an important role in pregnancies with positive outcomes (Parsa et al. 2012).

Fully immunized children (receiving the BCG, measles, or MMR vaccines, three DPT vaccinations, and three doses of polio vaccine) reached 94.0% in 2014 (UNICEF 2016a). The rate of infants (percentage of 1-year-olds) lacking measles immunization dropped to 1.0% in 2015. Similarly, the rate of infants lacking DTP immunization was reduced to 1.0% (United Nations Development Programme 2016a). In addition, the coverage of HBV vaccination of infantile vaccination has been very high in Iran (Lankarani et al. 2013).

In 2010, approximately 95% of the population had access to primary health care (Goudarzi et al. 2011). The physician density in Iran increased from 0.89 physicians per 1000 population in 2010 to 1.49 physicians per 1000 population in 2014, lower than the worldwide rate of 1.85 physicians per 1000 (World Bank 2018a) (Fig. 5.3 and Table 5.2). Hospital bed density was about 0.1 beds per 1000 population in 2012 (World Health Organization 2016). Iran has succeeded in reducing non-communicable diseases, improving maternal health, and fighting HIV/AIDS, smallpox, polio, malaria, and other communicable diseases. It is worth noting that there were no reported deaths related to malaria in Iran in 2015 due to the government's active policy to eliminate the disease (University of California San Francisco Global Health Group 2015).

Health improvement in Iran is also represented in the indicator that in 2015, 96.2% of the population in Iran (97.7% in urban locations and 92.1% in rural communities) had access to safe and improved water sources. Comparably, 90% of the Iranian population (92.8% urban and 82.3% rural) had access to sanitary systems. Primary health care units and centers numbered about 3.1 per 10,000 people. The population with access to local health services was 100% in urban settings and 95% in rural communities (Goudarzi et al. 2011) (Table 5.2).

Religious charities and private or non-governmental institutions (*bonyads*) participate in providing medical and rehabilitation services for the disabled, low-income groups, and rural dwellers (Saeidi 2009). All in all, formal and informal health systems in Iran formulate, implement, and monitor their policies and programs in line with promoting universal health coverage goals (UNESCO 2017).

5.3.2.2 Educational Well-Being in Iran

This section provides information on driver indicators of learning, which lend insight into the quality of educational provision in Iran. After the 1979 revolution, the most important change was the Islamization of the educational system. The Ministry of Education is currently responsible for the general formal, public, and free education in all domains of education, while the Ministry of Science, Research and Technology is responsible for the higher education (for non-medical universities).

Iran's education policy of "Vision 2025" seeks to establish "an education system capable of materializing *hayate tayyebah* (the ideal Islamic life), universal justice and Islamic-Iranian civilization" (Ministry of Education, Islamic Republic of Iran 2011: 6). It is worth pointing out that the private sector, supervised by the government or the Ministry of Education, participates in education for which it charges high tuition fees. The private sector manages the non-government schools whose number increased from 2000 schools in the 1990s to 13,893 schools in 2009–2010 reaching about 11% of all the country's schools and educating 1,100,000 students (Arani et al. 2015).

Iran has increased education expenditures from 2.8% of the total GDP in 2014 to 3.76% of the total GDP in 2016, a substantial increase in two years. This increase comprised 19.3% of total government expenditures in 2016 (UNESCO 2018b). The distribution of expenditures on students' education has varied based on the level of education (Fig. 5.5). For example, the government expenditure per student in 2015 was classified as follows: $1363 for a student enrolled in a primary school; $2593.57 for a student enrolled in a secondary school; and, $2393.19 for a student enrolled in a university (UNESCO 2018b).

The education system in Iran is divided into two main levels, primary education and high school education. According to the Ministry of Education, access to preprimary education among 5-year-old children has increased from 30% in 2000 to 55% in 2011. This improvement has been most significant in rural areas (United Nations Development Assistance Framework 2015). Compulsory education in Iran lasts 8 years, from age 6 to age 13 and within the following categories: primary (5 years, ages 6–10), lower secondary (3 years, ages 11–13) and upper secondary (4 years, ages 14–17). The primary school dropout rate was 3.8% of primary school cohorts in 2015 (UNESCO 2018b). Schools are divided by gender, and there are separate schools for boys and girls up to the end of secondary education (Arani et al. 2015) (Fig. 5.6). The government has made significant progress in training teachers to support quality education in all primary schools. By 2015, 100% of the teachers had training in education and the pupil-teacher ratio in primary schools was 26.77 pupils per teacher (UNESCO 2018b; United Nations Development Programme 2016b) (Fig. 5.6).

The Iranian government cooperates with international organizations such as the United Nations, UNICEF, and UNESCO to further develop its educational system. For instance, the UNESCO is currently supporting Iran in its efforts to achieve inclusive and quality education and promote lifelong learning opportunities for all, in the areas of education statistics, analysis, and reporting; literacy and lifelong learning; technical and vocational education and training; education for sustainable development; and ICT in education (UNESCO 2017). School is viewed as a hub for the country's general formal education system and a place for acquisition of developmental experience. The government of Iran has established education programs adopting Western curricula in the fields of science and technology. It is to be noted that despite Iran's acceptance of the institutional characteristics of Western education, particularly in higher education or universities, it attempts to maintain its religious-cultural norms (Sakurai 2017). Iran achieved a score of 3.5 (7 = high) and was globally ranked 113 (out of 138 countries) on the indicator of "Internet access in schools" (Fig. 5.7). Comparably, Iran was ranked 65 and 97 worldwide on the indicators of the "quality of primary education" and "quality of the higher education," respectively, in the 2015–2016 *Global Competitiveness Index* (World Economic Forum 2017) (Table 5.3).

As is the case in Egypt, teaching techniques in Iran need to be improved. Education policies suggest reducing the state monopoly of educational curricula and textbook production as well as employing professionalized teaching forces with higher salaries differentiated by mandatory relicensing (Heyneman 1997).

5.3.2.3 Economic Well-Being in Iran

Iran is the second largest economy in the MENA region after Saudi Arabia, with an estimated GDP of $412.2 billion in 2016. Iran's natural gas and oil reserves are, respectively, the second and fourth largest worldwide. The Iranian government has implemented a major reform policy of its subsidy program on key staples such as petroleum products, electricity, water, and bread, which has resulted in sufficient progress in the effectiveness of expenditures and economic activities (Central Intelligence Agency 2018). According to the *Global Competitiveness Report* 2015–2016, Iran was globally ranked 76 (out of 138 countries) (World Economic Forum 2017) (Fig. 5.8).

Despite the dominance of the oil sector, there are some signs of dynamism in the non-oil sectors as well. The domestic banking sector is well developed and financial inclusion is high, with 92% of people aged 15 years and more having a bank account (World Bank 2017b). Figure 5.8 shows that the driver of "market size" in Iran is large, globally ranked 19. Similarly, both input indicators of infrastructure and macroeconomic environment are improving, achieving global rankings of 59 and 72, respectively. On the indicators of "institution" and "innovation," Iran, within the lower half of the global rankings, was ranked 90 and 89, respectively (World Economic Forum 2017).

The general government final consumption expenditure of Iran's total GDP was 10.7%, which was lower than the worldwide average of 16.4%. It is worth noting that the general government final consumption expenditure refers to government spending on goods and services aimed at satisfying the individual and collective needs of members of the country (World Bank 2017b). The employment-to-population ratio for those aged 15 and older was 39.9% in 2015. The labor force participation rate for those aged 15 and older was 44.5%, whereas child labor (ages 5–14) was 11.0%. However, the participation of women in economic activity and the labor force in Iran is low compared to that of men. For instance, the labor force participation rate of the female population was 16.2% (ages 15 and older), whereas the labor force participation rate of the male population was 72.7% (ages 15 and older). Old-age pension recipients comprised 26.4% of the statutory pension-age population (United Nations Development Programme 2016a).

According to the 5-year development plan for the 2016–2021 period, Iran predicts an annual economic growth rate of 8%. Reforms of state-owned enterprises, the financial and banking sector, and the allocation and management of oil revenues are among the main priorities of the government (World Bank 2017b).

The government performance may be used as a significant driver impacting quality of life and well-being. For example, Table 5.5 shows that Iran is globally ranked 9 (and regionally ranked 1) on the input indicator of "government debt." In addition, Iran achieved an upper half global ranking of 52 on the indicator of "public trust in politicians" (World Economic Forum 2017) (Fig. 5.12). Despite the improved economy due to the use and sale of petroleum products and despite the fact that the Iranian government has used a public policy to reform its subsidy program on critical staples (World Bank 2017b) (Fig. 5.8), Iran still faces problems in certain aspects of government performance. The *Global Competitiveness Report* of 2015–2016 shows that Iran was globally ranked 116, 82 and 97, respectively, on the indicators of "transparency of government policy making," "wastefulness of government spending," and "burden of government regulation" (world Economic Forum 2017: 207) (Figs. 5.9, 5.10).

5.3.2.4 Communication and Technology in Iran

According to the *Networked Readiness Index* 2015, rating nations' deployment of ICT, Iran was globally ranked 96 (out of 139 countries) and 5 among the selected MENA countries. For the domain of "ICT use and government efficiency," Iran was globally ranked 63 and among the selected MENA countries, Iran was ranked 4. However, concerning the domain of the "availability of latest technologies," Iran underperformed with a rank of 111 worldwide and 5 among the selected MENA countries (World Economic Forum 2016) (Table 5.4).

5.3.2.5 Religious Tolerance and Political/Human Rights in Iran

Iran, a post-revolutionary state offering a model for a form of Islamization from the top (Eickelman 1992), is dominated by religiously oriented Shi'i clerics who mediate between the hidden Imam and the common Shi'a, who, in turn, seek guidance from the *marja'* or source of emulation (el-Aswad 2012: 60–62). According to the *Social Progress Index* (2017), Iran performed moderately on the indicator of religious tolerance with a score of 2 out of 4, but it did not perform well on the indicator of freedom of religion, recording a grade of 1 out 4 (1 = low). Iran, with a score of 7 out of 40 (40 = full rights), underperformed on the indicator of political rights. (Figure 5.11). It is worth noting that in Iran women's political activities are more difficult for the regime to suppress or control because it occurs outside of the formally recognized public sphere and women's informal economic activity is one of the primary drivers of political and social change (Eickelman 2008). Iran did not perform well on the indicator of political terror, scoring 3.5 out of 5 (5 = high). Further, Iran drastically underperformed on the indicator of freedom of expression, with a grade of 2 out of 16 (16 = full freedom) (Table 5.5). Iran has restrictive political systems or residues of prior systems that have deviated from democratic systems (Social Progress Index 2017). On the indicator of the level of violent crime, Iran performed well or evidenced less violent crime, achieving 2 out of 5 (5 = high); however, Iran performed within the lower half of the rankings on the indicator of "corruption," scoring 29 out of 100 (100 = low) (Fig. 5.12).

Iran's political culture has a critical impact on their public policy process. Iran regards the government of a qualified scholar ('*ālim*) or jurist (Arabic: *wilāyat al-faqiah*, Persian: *vilāyat-e faqīh*) as an ideal form of government until the appearance of the hidden imam (al-Mahdi) of the Twelver Shi'ism (el-Aswad 2010; Halm 2007; Louër 2008). The other important aspect of Iran's culture is the economic and political role stipulated by the 1979 Iranian constitution according to which family is "the fundamental unit of the Islamic society" (Eickelman and Piscatori 1996: 83).

5.3.3 Key Drivers in Israel

I discuss in this section key drivers of well-being in relation to health, education, economic well-being, communication technology, religious tolerance, and political right in Israel.

5.3.3.1 Health Well-Being in Israel

Israel has an effective primary care system, based on an accessible and well-managed network of community clinics, forming a significant driver of positive health outcomes in the country. The Israeli health care system is contingent on the National Health Insurance Law of 1995, which mandates all citizens resident in the country to join one of four official non-profit health insurance organizations known as Sick Funds. In addition to participating in one of the four compulsory health organizations, there are private health insurance plans that citizens may opt for (Organization for Economic Cooperation and Development 2015a).

In Israel, government social spending for 2016 constituted 57% of total government expenditures distributed as follows: 14% for health, 15% for education, and 28% for social welfare (Gal and Madhala 2017). In 2015, total health expenditure (public and private) in Israel was 7.7% of the GDP. Public or government health expenditure reached 4.8% of Israel's total GDP (United Nations Development Programme 2016a; World Health Organization 2017). The health spending per capita (PPP) in Israel was $2722 in 2015, highest among the selected MENA countries (Figs. 5.1, 5.2). The government health spending was 61.5% of total health spending, while out-of-pocket spending reached 27.3% of total health spending. Prepaid private spending was 11.2% of total health spending. The annualized rate of change in total health spending per capita for 1995–2014 was 1.9% (Financing Global Health 2016) (Table 5.1).

The main public health service that is included in the National Health Insurance benefits package is the preventive care clinics for young children and pregnant women (Rosen et al. 2015). Mandatory paid maternity leave is 98 days, giving mothers enough time for recovery and nursing (United Nations Development Programme 2016a). In Israel, fully immunized children (receiving BCG, measles, or MMR vaccination, three DPT vaccinations, and three doses of polio vaccine) reached 94.6% in 2014 (UNICEF 2016a). However, the problem of child immunization is still of concern in Israel. In 2015, 5% of infants (1-year-olds) lacked DTP immunization, whereas 4% lacked measles immunization (United Nations Development Programme 2016a) (Table 5.2).

In terms of the provision of medical personnel and facilities, physician density in Israel reached 3.62 physicians per 1000 people in 2014, surpassing the worldwide rate of 1.85 physicians per 1000 people according to the World Health Organization (2018); hospital bed density was about 3.3 beds per 1000 people in 2012 (Fig. 5.3). Furthermore, other health-related services, such as water treatments, are efficiently being provided. Israel has established innovative water treatment technologies for drinking water and wastewater recycling (Organization for Economic Cooperation and Development 2015a). Access to both improved drinking water sources and sanitation facilities is currently 100% reliable and secured. Around 80% of Israelis expressed their satisfaction with their health in 2013 (Organization for Economic Cooperation and Development 2015a) (Fig. 5.4).

Lifestyle factors also play a role, because Israelis generally have healthy lifestyle behaviors. They consume less sugar and alcohol, more fruits and vegetables, and are less likely to be smokers or obese (Organization for Economic Cooperation and Development 2015a). Despite an overall strong performance in the area of health, gaps in health care are widening as the privatization of health care rapidly increases (Gabbay 2016). For example, Arabs in Israel had significantly lower life expectancy (3 years less in the case of men, 3.4 years less in the case of women) in 2013 and higher rates of respiratory disease, diabetes, heart disease, and cancer, as well as higher rates of child and infant mortality than Jews. These differences reflect socioeconomic and cultural inequality or differences between communities in Israel that need to be effectively addressed (Organization for Economic Cooperation and Development 2015a).

5.3.3.2 Educational Well-Being in Israel

This subsection aims to show the efforts of the Israeli government to improve education through implementing specific drivers and policies in terms of governance, funding, schooling levels, preparing students for the future, training of teachers, and quality of instruction. The education system in Israel is managed by the central government, through the Ministry of Education, the Ministry of Finance, and local governments. However, the Ministry of Education determines education policy and is responsible for and oversees Israel's educational system including kindergartens, schools, higher education, and informal education (Ministry of Education, Israel 2018).

Since 2011, the Israeli government has subsidized public education for children ages 3–5 and has made education compulsory for those ages 5–17, making Israel's period of compulsory education one of the longest in the world (Organization for Economic Cooperation and Development 2016a). Classroom size is a key measure of academic quality. In Israel, the average classroom size is 27 at the primary level and 28 at the lower secondary level (Fig. 5.6). Comparatively, the pupil-teacher ratio for primary school is 13 students per teacher. Increasing teacher salaries will help schools recruit and retain the highly qualified teachers needed to offer all students a high-quality education (Walker 2012). In Israel, teachers of primary and secondary education have salaries comparable to those of similarly educated professionals (Organization for Economic Cooperation and Development 2015a). Higher education is provided by 63 higher education institutions, universities, academic colleges, and teacher-training colleges. Around 46% of Israelis ages 25 to 34 years have attained tertiary education, whereas 47% of the older Israeli generation (those aged 55 to 64 years) have attained tertiary or higher education (Organization for Economic Cooperation and Development 2016a).

Funding for schools is mostly provided by national and local governments. To be more specific, public expenditure on education includes government spending on educational institutions (both public and private), education administration as well as subsidies for private entities, including students, households, and other private agencies (UNESCO 2018c). As shown in Table 5.3, education expenditures deceased from 6.19% of the Israeli GDP in 2000 to 5.74% in 2014. However, public spending on education reached 14.28% of government expenditure in 2014 (World Bank 2018b). Government expenditure per student (in PPP$) in 2014 was distributed as follows: $7273 per student in primary education; $6235.09 per student in secondary education; and $6658.14 per student in tertiary education (UNESCO 2018c) (Fig. 5.5). Nevertheless, "Schools in the Arab education stream tend to be underfunded, as they are often located in less affluent areas…more affluent local governments can provide up to 10–20 times higher funding per student for schools than less affluent local governments" (Organization for Economic Cooperation and Development 2016a: 16).

Education policy was implemented in 2014/15 to support underperforming and disadvantaged students, including new immigrants, Arab-speaking minorities, and students of low socioeconomic status. The policy comprised an increase in the active usage of information technology including computers and the Internet, and an expansion in the allocation of special care hours for the disadvantaged population in primary and lower secondary school (Organization for Economic Cooperation and Development 2016a). According to the *Global Competitiveness Report* 2015–2016, Israel performed relatively well, achieving a score of 5.3 (7 = high) and was globally ranked 27 (out of 138 countries) on the indicator of "Internet access in schools" (World Economic Forum 2017). In the meantime, Israel was globally ranked 45 and 24 on the indicators of "quality of primary education," and "quality of the higher education," respectively (World Economic Forum 2017) (Fig. 5.7). However, Israel needs to expand and strengthen its provision of vocational education and training in order to improve transition to the labor market (Organization for Economic Cooperation and Development 2016a).

It is worth noting that Israel has a heterogeneous education system. From primary to upper secondary level, students are generally arranged into four main education streams of schools, three for the Hebrew-speaking community, including secular, religious, and ultra-orthodox, and one for the Arabic-speaking community such as the Arab, Druze, and Bedouin minorities (Organization for Economic Cooperation and Development 2016a). The problem here is that the education system is split in Israel, with achievement lower among orthodox-school and Arab-Israeli pupils (Organization for Economic Cooperation and Development 2016a; Sustainable Governance Indicators 2016). To be more specific, there are growing divisions or gaps in income, education, and civil rights between Arab-Palestinians and Israelis as well as between Ashkenazi Jews, those of American and European origins, and Mizrachi Jews, those from Arab countries (Cochran 2017; Leavy 2010; Nuseibeh 2016). Furthermore, educational achievements among the poor are in general very small and meager (Gabbay 2016). "Facing a lack of qualified teachers in all subjects, Israel needs to attract quality candidates to the profession and further improve teaching conditions" (Organization for Economic Cooperation and Development 2016a: 4) for all students.

5.3.3.3 Economic Well-Being in Israel

The Israeli economic and social policies have been very stable over the past decade. Israel managed to reduce its national debt from 100% of the GDP to 65% (1% being worth about $28.1 billion). It also reduced the tax burden by 4.5% of the GDP. Exports and imports improved, comprising 59.4% of Israel's total GDP (United Nations Development Programme 2016b). The employment-to-population ratio (for those ages 15 and older) in Israel has risen significantly, improving from 51.90% in 1990 to 60.8% in 2015, and the labor force participation rate reached 64.0% in 2015 (United Nations Development Programme 2016a). In addition, efforts on the part of recent governments to address social problems and ill-being have focused mainly on reducing the cost of living, especially with regard to housing, by encouraging free market competition and other price-lowering measures (Gal and Madhala 2017).

When assessing the global economic status of Israel, the *Global Competitiveness Report* (2015–2016) indicated that Israel had a global rank of 24 out of 138 countries. In 2015, Israel performed very well on the input indicators of "innovation," "infrastructure," and "institutions," achieving outstanding global ranks of 2, 28, and 31, respectively. By the same token, Israel achieved global ranks of 48 and 57, respectively, on the domains of "macroeconomic environment" and "market size" (World Economic Forum 2017) (Fig. 5.8).

In terms of government performance, Fig. 5.9 shows that Israel performed relatively well, achieving worldwide ranks of 39, 51, and 47 on the indicators of "transparency of government policymaking," "public trust in politicians," and "burden of government regulation," respectively. However, Israel did not perform within the expected range on the indicators of "government debt," globally ranked 96, and "wastefulness of government spending," with a worldwide rank of 78 (World Economic Forum 2017) (Fig. 5.10). These indicators measuring the performance of the government can be used to assist policy makers in proposing initiatives and public policies. A study dealing with well-being in Israel, conducted by the Organization for Economic Cooperation and Development (2015a), stated that, although "the economy performs well on key macro-economic indicators such as GDP growth, the affluence generated by certain sectors of economy has not benefitted at all, and poverty and inequality levels are high."

Overall, despite the fact that Israel's economic climate has improved, as reflected in declining unemployment rates and securing a higher GDP, "Israeli policymakers have made no major effort to reduce inequality or address social ills, whether through substantially increased social spending or a change in social policy direction" (Gal and Madhala 2017: 2). One of the possible social policies for the policy makers is to change the system of allocations from "priority" communities to underserved groups as well as to the population as a whole (Gabbay 2016).

5.3.3.4 Communication and Technology in Israel

A comprehensive assessment of well-being in a given country must embrace how that country utilizes technology to improve the quality of life of its people (Sirgy et al. 2017). Israel, often characterized as a "start-up nation," has a vibrant high-tech domain (Organization for Economic Cooperation and Development 2015a). Israel has shown an upward trend in advanced technologies. According to the Networked Readiness Index 2015, measuring countries' utilization of ICT, Israel was globally ranked 21 (out of 139 countries) and first among the selected MENA countries. However, for the domain of "ICT use and government efficiency," Israel was globally ranked 32 and among the selected MENA countries, it ranked second to the United Arab Emirates (UAE). Concerning the domain of the "availability of latest technologies," Israel performed well, achieving a rank of 8 worldwide and first among the selected MENA countries (World Economic Forum 2016) (Table 5.4).

5.3.3.5 Religious Tolerance and Political/Human Rights in Israel

According to the Social Progress Index (2017), Israel drastically underperformed on the indicator of "religious tolerance," scoring 1 out of 4 (1 = low), ranking 121 out of 128 countries. Israel also scored low on the indicator of "freedom of religion" with a grade of 2 out 4 (1 = low) (Fig. 5.11).

Israel, with a score of 36 out of 40 (40 = full rights), performed within the expected range on the indicator of political rights; however, Israel lagged significantly on parameters of personal freedom and choice as well as tolerance and inclusion (Social Progress Index 2017) (Table 5.5). Israel, within the upper half, ranked 61 out of 128 countries on the indicators of freedom of expression with a grade of 12 out of 16 (16 = full freedom). Israel performed within the lower half of the rankings on indicators of "level of violent crime" and "political terror," achieving 2 out of 5 (5 = high) in both categories. However, Israel performed within the expected range on the indicator of corruption, achieving 64 out of 100 (100 = low) (Social Progress Index 2017) (Fig. 5.12).

5.3.4 Key Drivers in Tunisia

I discuss in this section the key drivers of well-being in relation to health, education, economic well-being, communication technology, religious tolerance, and political right in Tunisia.

5.3.4.1 Health Well-Being in Tunisia

The main goal here is to determine the most important factors affecting health well-being as an essential driver of the overall well-being and quality of life in Tunisia. The Tunisian health care systems is administered by the Ministry of Public Health. Tunisia's health care system has been the focus of continued public initiatives managing public and private sectors including hospitals and health centers established nationwide. Tunisia's well-developed physical infrastructure has played an important role in the country's well-being. The main objective of Tunisia's health care system is to provide the Tunisian citizens with free and reliable health care.

Health expenditures are anticipated to increase due to such factors as the rapid growth of population, rising income, increasing health awareness, and demand for new health technologies and services. Table 5.1 shows that health spending per capita (PPP$) in Tunisia was around $791.0 in 2015. Total health expenditure (public and private) in 2014 was 7.0% of the GDP, ranking second out of the six MENA countries. The government health spending was 57.2% of total health spending, whereas out of pocket spending reached 38.1% per total health spending. The annualized rate of change in total health spending per capita for 1995–2014 was 3.5% (Financing Global Health 2016) (Figs. 5.1, 5.2). Social health insurance as a share of current health expenditure in Tunisia increased from 18.1% in 2001 to 32.3% in 2015, growing at an average annual rate of 5.15% (World Data Atlas 2018c).

Access to prenatal care is an important part of primary health care serving pregnant women. The rate of pregnant women receiving prenatal care improved from 91.5% in 2000 to 98.1% in 2012 (World Bank 2018a). For working women, there should be an increase in child-related leave entitlements, which are presently as low as 30 days of paid maternity leave (less than that of other selected MENA countries), with no unpaid-leave entitlement (Organization for Economic Cooperation and Development 2015b).

The provision of vaccinations or immunizations is an important driver for maintaining children or people's overall well-being. In Tunisia, fully immunized children (receiving BCG, measles, or MMR vaccination, three DPT vaccinations, and three doses of polio vaccine) reached 93.0% in 2014 (UNICEF 2016a). Further health-related data revealed that infants (percentage of 1-year-olds) lacking measles immunization in 2015 reached 2.0%, whereas infants lacking DTP immunization in 2015 also reached 2.0% (United Nations Development Programme 2016a).

The country ranks highly in terms of the availability of basic services. For instance, in 2015, there were 1.289 physicians per 1000 people compared to 0.537 per 1000 people in 1990 and 0.676 per 1000 people in 2000 (World Bank 2018b) (Fig. 5.3). About 99.5% of households had access to electricity, 94% to sanitation facilities, and more than 97% to improved drinking water in 2014 (Organization for Economic Cooperation and Development 2015b) (Fig. 5.4).

As a whole, Tunisia's health care system depends on its relatively stable foundation, boosting private sector, and qualified workforce. In addition, the government has focused on policies aimed at identifying medium- to long-term reform measures that will reduce health inequalities and improve the system's responses to the evolving demographic and epidemiologic situation (Oxford Business Group 2016). However, according to the World Health Organization (2017), health system reform is needed in order to implement an integrated approach focusing on primary care, prevention, and provision of palliative care in order to better respond to the increase in non-communicable diseases.

5.3.4.2 Educational Well-Being in Tunisia

Education has become one of the important input indicators of happiness and high quality of life. And, access to high-quality education is a driver of other domains of well-being such as income, health, employment, and social status (Layard 2005; Michalos 2007). The Tunisian government considers the achievement of universal education a top priority.

The Ministry of Education, Republic of Tunisia (2018) is responsible for public and private education including preschool, primary, and secondary levels. The Ministry of Higher Education, Scientific Research and Technology is responsible for the tertiary or university level education. Government expenditure on education was 6.60% of Tunisia's total GDP, higher than that of the selected MENA countries, and the education expenditure was 22.9% of the total government expenditure in 2015 (UNESCO 2018d). Government expenditure per student (in PPP$) is classified as follows: $1674.06 for each student enrolled in primary education as of 2008; $6059.65 for each student enrolled in secondary school as of 2015; and $6330.63 for each student enrolled in tertiary education as of 2015 (UNESCO 2018d) (Fig. 5.5).

Compulsory education lasts 9 years including 6 years of primary school, 3 years of preparatory (lower secondary), and 4 years of upper secondary school. The number of primary school teachers who were trained to teach scored high, reaching 100%. The student-teacher ratio has decreased to 17 pupils per teacher (United Nations Development Programme 2016a) (Fig. 5.6). Furthermore, the Ministry of Education, with the UNICEF support, implemented a policy of "second chance" education for children dropping out of school, resulting in the continuation of 9589 children in school in 2016, reducing the dropout rate by 10% (UNICEF 2016b). The Tunisian government plans, within a general education policy, to include preschool (between 3 and 5 years of age) based on the viewpoint that the years preceding primary education are crucial for children's development (UNICEF 2015b).

Although Tunisia has continued to prioritize investment in education, it has paid too little attention to the requirements of the labor market. This approach has led to a mismatch between qualifications and the needs of the employment market. The authorities have to continue renovating Tunisia's higher education system by providing reliable career guidance and ensuring better employability for new graduates (Oxford Business Group 2016).

The Tunisian government is currently working to introduce a series of reforms as part of the Strategic Plan for the Education Sector 2016–20. The 5-year plan aims to improve the quality of teaching, develop teachers' training, promote research and innovation, foster good governance, and optimize resource management. To improve the quality of teaching and learning, Tunisia has invested in digital technology to support education. However, there seems to be a need to encourage vocational education and training to increase employment among graduates (Organization for Economic Cooperation and Development 2015b).

According to the *Global Competitiveness Report* 2015–2016, Tunisia achieved 3.5 (7 = high) and was ranked 112 worldwide on the indicator of "Internet access in schools." It is worth noting that Tunisia was also globally ranked 85 and 107 on the indicators of the "quality of primary education" and "quality of the higher education," respectively (World Economic Forum 2017) (Fig. 5.7). Overall, the government needs to improve the quality of education at all levels through multiple interventions including improved facilities, updated curricula, increased collaboration among stakeholders, enhanced support for weaker and disabled students, and provision of reliable transport and school food options.

5.3.4.3 Economic Well-Being in Tunisia

Political unrest during 2011 and terrorist attacks against the tourism sector have had a negative impact on the economy (Central Intelligence Agency 2018). Despite the political turmoil, the government has managed to improve the economy by following a progressive economic policy of bolstering foreign investment, tourism, and exports, thereby improving well-being and living standards. Both exports and imports increased, reaching 102.1% of the total GDP in 2015. Important exports included petroleum products, textiles and apparel, food products, and phosphates (United Nations Development Programme, Tunisia 2016a). Other industries driving the Tunisian economy include services (63.5% of the total GDP), industry (25.9% of the total GDP), agriculture (10% of the total GDP), and remittances (5.46% of the total GDP) (Central Intelligence Agency 2018).

The employment-to-population ratio in Tunisia has grown from 38.10% in 1997 to 40.6% in 2015. Between 2010 and 2013, employment in the general government increased by 26% because wage and benefit levels are substantially higher for public employees than for private ones (Organization for Economic Cooperation and Development 2015b). The labor force participation rate (for people ages 15 and older) improved from 39.70% in 2000 to 47.7% in 2015. Employment in services reached 51.5% of the total employment, whereas employment in agriculture reached 14.8% (International Labor Organization 2017; United Nations Development Programme 2016a). However, active labor market policies should be better targeted and vocational and educational training strengthened (Organization for Economic Cooperation and Development 2015b).

When assessing the global economic status of Tunisia, the Global Competitiveness Report (2015–2016) indicated that Tunisia had a global rank of 95 out of 138 countries. As shown in Fig. 5.8, Tunisia performed relatively well on input indicators of "market size," "institutions," and "infrastructure," achieving global ranks of 69, 78, and 83, respectively. However, on indicators of "innovation" and macroeconomic environment" Tunisian scored low with global ranks of 99 and 104, respectively (World Economic Forum 2017).

Tunisia relies on price subsidies for energy and food products to protect poor households' purchasing power (Organization for Economic Cooperation and Development 2015b). There have been progressive policies in Tunisia aimed at reducing the gender gap, particularly in the private sector, strengthening public awareness of antidiscrimination laws, promoting pay transparency, and improving enforcement of equal-pay provisions (Organization for Economic Cooperation and Development 2015b).

According to the *Global Competitiveness Report* of 2015–2016, Tunisia, within the upper half of the global rankings, was ranked 63 and 65 on the indicators of "public trust in politicians" and "wastefulness of government spending," respectively. Nonetheless, Tunisia faces problems that might hinder the realization of well-being (Fig. 5.9). These problems relate to the indicators of "burden of government regulation," globally ranked 104, "transparency of government policymaking," ranked 91, and "government debt," with a worldwide rank of 81 (World Economic Forum 2017) (Fig. 5.10).

Although overall the economy of Tunisia has improved, unemployment is still high at 15% (World Bank 2016), and the inflation rate, higher than those of all of the selected MENA countries, reached 12.9% in 2016 and ranked 109 out of 138 countries globally (World Economic Forum 2017). As is the case with most MENA countries, the Tunisian government is highly centralized. The recommendation here is that decentralization may produce positive results and bring governance closer to the people and thereby enhance their happiness and overall well-being.

5.3.4.4 Communication and Technology in Tunisia

Tunisia has shown progress with communication technologies. According to the Networked Readiness Index 2015, measuring the propensity for countries to utilize the opportunities offered by ICT, Tunisia was globally ranked 81 (out of 139 countries) and 6 (or the last) among the selected MENA countries. For the domain of "ICT use and government efficiency," Tunisia was globally ranked 92 and 5 among the selected countries. Concerning the domain of the "availability of latest technologies," Tunisia achieved a global rank of 83 worldwide and 4 among the selected MENA countries (World Economic Forum 2016). These data may suggest that although Tunisia has access to technology, it may not have yet maximized its use for governmental and personal opportunities (Table 5.4).

5.3.4.5 Religious Tolerance and Political/Human Rights in Tunisia

According to the Social Progress Index (2017), Tunisia underperformed on the indicator of religious tolerance with a score of 2 out of 4 as well as on the indicator of freedom of religion with a score of 2 out of 4 (1 = low) (Fig. 5.11). Tunisia scored very high on the indicator for political rights, achieving 36 out of 40 (40 = full rights). On the indicator of freedom of expression, Tunisia again achieved a high score of 13 out of 16 (16 = high) (Fig. 5.12). On the indicator of the level of violent crime, Tunisia performed within the expected range, achieving a score of 2 out of 5 (5 = high). Similarly,

Tunisia performed within expected ranges on indicators of political terror with a grade of 2 out 5 (5 = high) and of corruption with a grade of 41 out of 100 (100 = low) (Table 5.5).

5.3.5 *Key Drivers in Turkey*

I discuss in this section the key drivers of well-being in relation to health, education, economic well-being, communication technology, religious tolerance, and political right in Turkey.

5.3.5.1 Health Well-Being in Turkey

The Ministry of Health of Turkey is the main provider of health care in Turkey. In the last two decades, many public and private institutions have designed strategic plans in order to establish their missions and objectives. To be more specific, the Ministry of Health initiated the strategic plan for the years 2013–2017 in which past health achievements as well as future objectives in health care are documented (Ministry of Health of Turkey 2012). During the period 2003–2011, the Health Transformation Program in Turkey, initiated in 2003 to ensure efficient and equitable health service delivery, paid special attention to primary care services, particularly preventive health care and maternal-child health care services. In addition, comprehensive policies were implemented to raise health funds to prevent ill-health and premature deaths associated with non-communicable diseases (Ministry of Health of Turkey 2012).

The total health expenditure (public and private) in Turkey reached 5.4% of the GDP, whereas public health expenditures reached 4.2% of the GDP in 2014 (Figs. 5.1, 5.2). Government health spending was 78.4% of total health spending (highest among the selected MENA countries), whereas out of pocket spending reached 18.0% of total health spending. Meanwhile, the health spending per capita purchasing (PPP$) was $1040.0 in 2015, and prepaid private spending comprised 3.5% of total health spending. The annualized rate of change in total health spending per capita for 1995 to 2014 was 6.6%, highest among the selected MENA countries (Financing Global Health 2016) (Table 5.1 and Fig. 5.2).

The government of Turkey has made progress in health infrastructure and services. Hospital bed density improved, reaching 3 beds per 1000 people in 2012. The physician density increased from 0.94 physicians per 1000 people in 1990 to 1.44 physicians per 1000 people in 2000, and then to 1.75 physicians per 1000 people in 2014 (World Bank 2018d) (Fig. 5.3). In addition, 100% of the population had access to improved drinking water and 98.3% of the population had the benefits of sanitation facilities as of 2015 (Central Intelligence Agency 2018) (Fig. 5.4 and Table 5.2). According to the Strategic Plan 2013–2017, Turkey improved the health care services provided to the elderly and individuals with low income (Ministry of Health of Turkey 2012).

In 2011, a project entitled "Guest-Mom" was initiated to serve pregnant women and encourage them and their children to have their health checked regularly (Ministry of Health of Turkey 2012). Among other health initiatives and plans is the "Turkish Mental Health Action Plan," which established 50 community-based mental health services in 44 provinces in 2012 (Ministry of Health of Turkey 2012). Pregnant women receiving prenatal care reached 96.9% in 2013, improved from 62.2% in 1993 (World Bank 2018a). Mandatory paid maternity leave has been established at 112 days, beneficial for the mother and the child. Fully immunized children (receiving BCG, measles, or MMR vaccinations, three DPT vaccinations, and three doses of polio vaccine) reached 94.4.0% in 2014 (UNICEF 2015a). Comparably, infants (percentage of 1-year-olds) lacking measles immunization in 2015 reached 6.0%, whereas infants lacking DTP immunization reached 3.0% (United Nations Development Programme 2016a).

According to the Tenth Development Plan (2014–2018), the goals of health care include increasing the quality of life and life span of the citizens and ensuring their participation in the economic, social, and cultural life in a conscious, active manner. For this purpose, accessible, qualified, cost-effective, and sustainable health service delivery supported by evidence-based policies is essential (Republic of Turkey 2014). It is worthy to point out that tobacco use in Turkey is declining at unprecedented rates due to an aggressive smoking ban in public indoor and outdoor arenas and the provision of medical assistance to addicts (Daily Sabah 2016; Gürbüz 2017). The improvement of health care is reflected in the rate concerning the general satisfaction with health services in Turkey that reached 76% of the population in 2012 (Ministry of Health of Turkey 2012).

5.3.5.2 Educational Well-Being in Turkey

The education system in Turkey includes two major sectors: formal or public and informal or private. Formal education comprises preschool, which is voluntary and covers children ages 3–5, and primary, of which 8 years are compulsory covering the ages of 6 to 14. Secondary education (4 years) includes the options of mainly general and technical and vocational education and training. In 2012, there were about 67,000 schools in Turkey. Tertiary education consists of 2-year vocational colleges and/or

4-year universities (Organization for Economic Cooperation and Development 2013, 2016b).

Successful public policies depend largely on the ability of the government to coordinate policy design and implementation. In Turkey, increases in the recruitment and in-service training opportunities of teachers and in public resources allocated to education have been materialized. Government expenditure on education in Turkey was 4.77% of the GDP as of 2013. Education expenditure per student (in PPP$) in 2014 was allocated as follows: $3316.73 per student enrolled in primary education; $2599.56 per student enrolled in secondary school; and $5044.69 per student enrolled in tertiary education (UNESCO 2018e) (Table 5.3 and Fig. 5.5).

The Ministry of National Education, supported by other ministries and private sectors, has provided initiatives and education policies to advance all levels of education with special focus on basic compulsory education (Organization for Economic Cooperation and Development 2013). The pupil-teacher ratio of primary school decreased to 20 pupils per teacher, whereas the average classroom size was reduced to 23 students as of 2015 (United Nations Development Programme 2016a) (Fig. 5.6).

According to Turkey's Tenth Development Plan (2014–2018), the main goal of education policy is to raise happy and productive individuals who have critical and innovative thinking as well as to facilitate access to quality learning through strengthening lifelong learning infrastructure, applying advanced technology, and recruiting highly qualified teachers. Several educational goals, such as improving the quality of education by using technology, providing free textbooks and transportation for students, and increasing the rates of girls' enrollment at all levels of education have been realized (Republic of Turkey 2014). According to the *Global Competitiveness Index* 2015, Turkey scored 4.1 (7 = high) and was ranked 79 worldwide on the indicator of "Internet access in schools." However, as shown in Table 5.3, Turkey was globally ranked 105 and 104 on the indicators of the "quality of primary education" and "quality of the higher education," respectively (World Economic Forum 2017) (Fig. 5.7). Such measurements imply an urgent call for implementing more educational policies to improve the quality of education in Turkey.

5.3.5.3 Economic Well-Being in Turkey

Turkey has improved its economy by applying assertive policies boosting industry, foreign trade, exports, public services, and finance. Turkey's average annual growth was 6.7% in 2015. Exports and imports comprised 58.8% of Turkey's GDP; industry and agriculture made up 31.8% and 6.7% of the GDP, respectively. Turkey's general government final consumption expenditure in 2015 was 15.5% (United Nations Development Programme 2016a). Labor force participation rate in Turkey in 2015 was 50.3% (of those ages 15 and older). The employment-to-population ratio (of those ages 15 and older) increased from 40.70% in 2000 to 46.10% in 2015 (United Nations Development Programme 2016a).

Turkey has the potential for new breakthroughs in catching up with high income countries through its demographic characteristics, increased quality of labor, long-established industrialization experience, large domestic market, proximity to developed markets, and access to emerging markets (Republic of Turkey 2014). Turkey's assertive privatization policy managed to reduce state involvement in basic industry, banking, transport, power generation, and communication. Turkey's well-regulated financial markets and banking system helped the country survive the global financial crisis of 2008–2009 (Central Intelligence Agency 2018). Furthermore, Turkey managed to endure the challenges related to the influx of more than 3 million Syrian refugees in 2015–2016 that created new social, economic, and political demands, particularly in urban centers (United Nations High Commissioner for Refugees 2016).

In Turkey, one of the most important actions in the domain of policy issues was the introduction of the Family and Social Policies Ministry (in 2011), which is responsible for family affairs and social services as well as for alleviating poverty and helping the elderly, disabled, and socially disadvantaged groups. In 2013, 1.26% of Turkey's total GDP was allocated for social assistance spending, which was a highly elevated percentage compared to previous years (Gürbüz 2017). Old-age pension recipients increased, reaching 88.1% of the statutory pension-aged population (United Nations Development Programme 2016a).

Figure 5.8 shows that the market size in Turkey is ranked first regionally and 17 globally. Comparably, Turkey has shown moderate progress on the input indicators of infrastructure, institutions, macroeconomic environment, and innovation (World Economic Forum 2017).

Turkey performs relatively well on the domains of government debt (ranked globally 27), government spending (38), and transparency of government policy making (47). However, on the indicators of "public trust in politicians" and "burden of government regulation," Turkey achieved in the lower half, ranking 74 and 71, respectively (World Economic Forum 2017) (Figs. 5.9, 5.10).

This shortcoming in the performance of the government can be resolved through efficient policies and adequate reforms aimed at boosting flexibility and applying innovation and talent more effectively. For instance, the state might propose flexible policies to ease or alleviate governmental regulations and administrative requirements imposed on businessmen and other professionals in both public and private sectors.

5.3.5.4 Communication and Technology in Turkey

The ICT sector has become an important part of Turkey's economic and social well-being. According to the Networked Readiness Index 2015, which measures the propensity for countries to utilize the opportunities offered by ICT, Turkey ranked 48 globally (out of 139 countries) and 3 among the selected MENA countries. For the domain of "ICT use and government efficiency," Turkey ranked 43 globally and 3 among the selected countries. Concerning the domain of the "availability of latest technologies," Turkey achieved a global rank of 55 worldwide and 3 among the selected MENA countries (World Economic Forum 2016) (Table 5.4).

5.3.5.5 Religious Tolerance and Political/Human Rights in Turkey

Turkey is "a secularized, democratic Muslim state in which religious sentiment and practice pervade public life but do not eclipse it" (Eickelman 1992: 5). According to the Social Progress Index (2017), Turkey performed relatively well on the indicator of "religious tolerance," with a grade of 2 out of 4 (4 = high), but it underperformed on the indicator of "freedom of religion," with a score of 1 out 4 (1 = low, 4 = high) (Fig. 5.11). Further, Turkey performed within the lower half of the rankings on "political rights," scoring 18 out of 40 (40 = full rights). However, Turkey underperformed on the indicator of "political terror," with a grade of 3.5 out of 5 (5 = high) and on the indicator of "level of violent crime," with a score of 3 out of 5 (5 = high) (Table 5.5). Turkey drastically underperformed on the indicator of "freedom of expression," scoring 6 out of 16 (16 = full freedom). In addition, Turkey performed moderately on the indicator of "corruption," scoring 41 out of 100 (100 = low) (Fig. 5.12).

5.3.6 Key Drivers in the United Arab Emirates (UAE)

I discuss in this section the key drivers of well-being in relation to health, education, economic well-being, communication technology, religious tolerance, and political right in UAE.

5.3.6.1 Health Well-Being in the United Arab Emirates

According to the *Global Competitiveness Index* of 2015–2016, the UAE lead the MENA region in significant fields of well-being, achieving a worldwide rank of 16 out of 138 countries (World Economic Forum 2017). This achievement is mirrored in the performance indicators in the domains of health care, education, knowledge, economy, and governance declared in October 2014 by the "UAE Vision 2021 National Agenda" (United Arab Emirates 2014).

The United Arab Emirates Ministry of Health and Prevention, the main provider of health care in the UAE, is responsible for the implementation of health care policy. The mission is to enhance community health by providing comprehensive, innovative, and fair or equal health care services as per international standards. Health insurance, through public and private agencies, is mandatory for all residents in the UAE.

According to its health strategy (United Arab Emirates Ministry of Health and Prevention 2018), the Ministry of Health and Prevention is currently expanding health facilities and hospitals, health clinics, and medical centers in the seven emirates.

It is to be noted that health care in the UAE is regulated at the federal level as well as at the level of each constituent emirate. For instance, the health care sector in the emirate of Abu Dhabi is managed by the Department of Health in Abu Dhabi, known as the Health Authority Abu Dhabi (2018), whereas the health care sector in the emirate of Dubai is regulated by the Dubai Health Authority (2018). In 2002, the Dubai Healthcare City was launched to provide quality health care and serve as an integrated center of excellence for clinical and wellness services, medical education, and research in the Middle East.

The public policies in the UAE have succeeded in securing enough funds for supporting projects that facilitate good quality of life and well-being. The total health expenditure (public and private) reached 3.6% of the total GDP as of 2015. The public health expenditure of the UAE reached 2.6% of the total GDP in 2014 (World Health Organization 2017). The per capita (PPP$) health spending in the UAE was $2561.0 in 2015. The government health spending was 72.3% of total health spending (highest among the selected MENA countries), whereas out of pocket spending reached 17.8% of total health spending, the lowest among the selected MENA countries. Prepaid private spending comprised 9.9% of the total health spending in 2014 (Figs. 5.1, 5.2). The annualized rate of change in total health spending per capita for 1995–2014 was 0.4%, the lowest among the selected MENA countries (Financing Global Health 2016) (Table 5.1). The U.A.E.'s health expenditure reached a value of Arab Emirates Dirham (AED) 59.15 billion (US$16 billion) in 2016. This includes health care expenditures from all the seven emirates in addition to their contribution to the federal budget (United Arab Emirates Ministry of Health and Prevention 2018).

Over the past two decades, the UAE has been involved with a large-scale policy aimed at improving health care and health services. Health care provided to all residents, particularly child and maternal health services, has become a priority in the UAE. Pregnant women receiving prenatal care increased from 98.9% in 2004 to 100% in 2015 (World Health Organization 2016) (Table 5.2). The national neonatal screening program for newborn babies increased from 50% in 1998 to 95% in 2010, resulting in early detection and successful treatments. The mandatory paid maternity leave is 45 days. The UAE has made progress with the control and prevention of communicable diseases with a particular focus on immunization, surveillance, mandatory reporting, and effective treatment (Koornneef et al. 2017). Fully immunized children (receiving BCG, measles or MMR vaccination, three DPT vaccinations, and three doses of polio vaccine) reached 95.0% in 2014 (UNICEF 2015a). Infants (percentage of 1-year-olds) lacking measles immunization in 2015 reached 6.0%. A similar rate of 6.0% was recorded for infants lacking DTP immunization (United Nations Development Programme 2016a).

The UAE government implemented an operational policy to reduce rates of obesity that reached 34.5% of the population. In addition, the government carried out an operational policy to fight diabetes that reached 8.0% of the population in 2014 (World Health Organization 2016). The total number of hospital beds has more than doubled, reaching 2 beds per 1000 people in 2012 (Central Intelligence Agency 2018), and there has been almost a fivefold increase in the number of nurses and medical practitioners (Koornneef et al. 2017), reaching 1.56 physicians per 1000 people in 2014 (World Bank 2018d) (Fig. 5.3). The UAE government has improved other health services and infrastructure. Table 5.2 shows that the rate of the improved drinking water reached 99.6% of the population, whereas that of access to sanitation facilities increased to 98% of the population in 2015 (Central Intelligence Agency 2018) (Fig. 5.4). According to the *Global Competitiveness Index* 2015–2016, the UAE was globally ranked 10, scoring a grade of 6.7 (7 = high) on the indicator of the quality of the supply of electricity (World Economic Forum 2017).

5.3.6.2 Educational Well-Being in the United Arab Emirates

The educational system of the UAE is comparatively new, particularly since the establishment of the federation of the seven emirates in 1971. Education at primary and secondary levels is operated by both public and private sectors. About 60% of all students attend public schools, whereas 40% of student attend private schools (Bertelsmann Stiftung 2016).

The Ministry of Education is responsible for managing and funding public education including kindergarten (4–5 years old), primary schools (6–11 years old), preparatory schools (12–14 years old), and high schools (15–18 years old) as well as technical secondary schools that serve 12–18-year-old students. In 2005, the Abu Dhabi Education Council, working closely with the Ministry of Education, was founded to further develop education throughout the UAE. A training initiative called Tanmia was launched in January 2015, through which all public school teachers embarked on professional training as a means to improve the quality of teaching (Bertelsmann Stiftung 2016).

The United Arab Emirates' public spending on education as a share of GDP was 1.1% in 1997 (UNESCO 2018f) (Fig. 5.5). However, the 2014 federal budget allocated 49% for development projects focusing on education and health provisions. In 2016, 21.2% of the UAE budget (AED 48.5 billion, equivalent to $13.2 billion) was allocated for developing the education sector (Al Masah Capital 2016). The issue taken into consideration here is the small national population size compared to the strong GDP of the UAE. According to HSBC's Value of Education report in 2017, $99,378 was the average total amount spent by Emirati parents for one child from primary school to the undergraduate level (The National 2017). The percentage of primary school teachers trained to teach was 100% in 2015 and the pupil-teacher ratio of primary schools was 19 pupils per teacher (Fig. 5.6). Moreover, Emirati women maintain higher levels of education compared to men. For instance, the population with at least some secondary education among women was 77.4% (ages 25 and older), whereas that among men was 64.5% as of 2015 (United Nations Development Programme 2016a).

The Ministry of Education, in its attempts to ensure equal educational opportunities for all, is currently implementing a major education policy entitled the "Ministry of Education Strategic Plan 2017–2021." The plan is designed to elevate education to reach the level of a world-class education system by increasing proficiency in technology, introducing advanced education techniques, updating curricula, developing innovative skills, and strengthening self-learning abilities of students (United Arab Emirates Ministry of Education 2018). The UAE performed well, scoring 6.1 (7 = high) and was ranked 4 worldwide on the indicator of "Internet access in schools"

(Fig. 5.7). In addition, the UAE was globally ranked 10 and 12 out of 138 countries on the indicators of the "quality of the higher education" and "quality of primary education," respectively, in the 2015–2016 *Global Competitiveness Report* (World Economic Forum 2017) (Table 5.3).

The UAE has established international research collaborations with global education institutes and agencies such as the New York University in Abu Dhabi, the Paris-Sorbonne University Abu Dhabi, the Virginia Commonwealth University School of Business, to mention a few (Ahmed 2016). The Dubai Knowledge Village, launched in 2003, is currently hosting branches of reputable regional and international universities from Australia, Belgium, Canada, India, Iran, Ireland, Pakistan, Russia, and the United Kingdom. Each branch applies the programs, teaching methods, degrees, and accreditation identical to its homeland institute or university (Dubai Knowledge Village 2018). The Dubai International Academic City (2018), launched in April 2007, is the world's largest free zone dedicated to higher education; it currently serves over 24,000 students from around the world.

5.3.6.3 Economic Well-Being in the United Arab Emirates

The UAE is one of the leading oil producers of the world, and the government ensures that much of the revenue from hydrocarbon sales is used for the development of its country. The UAE has witnessed its GDP rise from $46 billion in 1995 to $418 billion in 2014, an increase of close to 1000% (Bertelsmann Stiftung 2016). The UAE, leading other the Gulf States, has implemented a policy of economic diversification by supporting non-oil revenues to be key contributory drivers to an enhanced economy (Al Masah Capital 2016, 2018).

In terms of its market economy, the UAE has continued its substantial growth supported by reform policies that provide a resilient institutional framework. The UAE's "Vision 2021" strategic policy sets the goal of becoming an economic, touristic, and commercial capital by emphasizing the building of a knowledge-based economy that supports innovation, entrepreneurship, and advances in research and development.

The UAE has pursued an economic liberalization strategy by boosting its capital market system and banking. More than 23 national banks, six GCC banks, and 22 foreign banks were operating in the country as of January 2013 (Bertelsmann Stiftung 2016). The UAE's general government final consumption expenditure in 2015 was 7.5%, and the average annual growth rate was 3.7%. The UAE was ranked 22 globally in 2015 by the World Bank. The country's free trade zones, which offer 100% foreign ownership and zero taxes, attract foreign investors (World Bank 2017c).

The UAE has enjoyed long-term economic security. Presently, citizens of the UAE enjoy tax-free income, free national housing for Emirati nationals who are economically unable to purchase houses, subsidized fuel, and lavish retirement plans funded by the government. On certain celebratory occasions, such as the Emirates National Day, the loans and debts of Emirati nationals are paid by the state (el-Aswad 2015). It is worth noting that on May 6, 2018, all serving and retired UAE government employees as well as employees of a privately owned cooperative retail chain and beneficiaries of social welfare services were paid a 1-month basic salary as a bonus for the occasion of the centennial anniversary of the late Sheikh Zayed, the founding leader of the UAE (Khaleej Times 2018; The National 2018).

The UAE leads the MENA region in the *Global Competitiveness Report* of 2015–2016, achieving a worldwide rank of 16 out of 138 countries. The UAE performs extremely well on the input indicators of "infrastructure" and "institutions," attaining global ranks of 4 and 7, respectively. As shown in Fig. 5.8, the UAE has shown remarkable progress in the domains of innovation, market size, and macroeconomic environment, achieving worldwide ranks of 25, 27, and 38, respectively (World Economic Forum 2017).

The degree of confidence that people have in the political system and government may serve as an indicator of the quality of their government's performance. A recent study has shown that there are strong linkages between smart government, happiness, and good governance (Yaghi and Al-Jenaibi 2018). The UAE achieved a high score of 5.6 (7 = high) and ranked 14 worldwidev on the indicator of "transparency of government policymaking." In addition, the UAE ranked 2 on indicators of both "public trust in politicians" and "wastefulness of government spending." On the indicator of "burden of government regulation," the UAE, ranked in the upper half of the global rankings, achieving a rank of 71 worldwide (World Economic Forum 2017) (Figs. 5.9, 5.10).

The UAE has adopted the most affluent social-public policies of the MENA countries, including welfare, health care, free public education, maternity leave, state pensions, permanent employment, and national security (Al Masah Capital 2016; Arabian Business 2016). Despite their outstanding public services, the UAE state needs to generate effective policies to lighten the burden of government regulations in dealing with public and privates sectors as well as with civil society.

5.3.6.4 Communication and Technology in the United Arab Emirates

Certain forms of cyber communication have become increasingly the most spectacular channels of communication and social interaction among the Emirati people (el-Aswad 2014a). According to the Networked Readiness Index 2015, measuring the propensity for countries to utilize ICT opportunities, the UAE was ranked 26 globally (out of 139 countries) and 2 among the selected MENA countries. For the domain of "ICT use and government efficiency," the UAE ranked first globally and first among the selected MENA countries. Concerning the domain of the "availability of latest technologies," the UAE achieved a global rank of 9 worldwide and 3 among the selected MENA countries (World Economic Forum 2016) (Table 5.4).

5.3.6.5 Religious Tolerance and Political/Human Rights in the United Arab Emirates

According to the Social Progress Index (2017), the UAE performed within expected ranges on indicators of "religious tolerance," with a grade of 3 out of 4 (4 = high), and "freedom of religion," with a score 3 out of 4 (4 = high) (Fig. 5.11). The UAE gravely underperformed on the indicator of "political rights," with a grade of 7 out of 40 (40 = full rights) and "freedom of expression" with a score of 4 out of 16 (16 = full freedom) (Fig. 5.12). The UAE underperformed on the indicators of "political terror," scoring 2.5 out of 5 (5 = high) and "level of violent crime" scoring 1 out of 5 (5 = high). Moreover, the Emirates performed within expected ranges on the indicator of corruption, scoring 66 out of 100 (100 = low) (Table 5.5).

5.4 Human Rights and Religious Tolerance: A Comparative Analysis

This section addresses seven indicators related to religion and human rights well-being in the selected MENA countries. For the domain of "religious tolerance," the UAE ranked in first place (with a score of 3 out of 4), followed by the other countries, whereas Israel ranked last (with a score of 1 out of 4; 1 = low). Concerning "freedom of religion," the UAE led, followed by Israel and Tunisia, then Iran, Turkey, and Egypt (Fig. 5.11). Regarding "freedom of expression," Tunisia ranked first (with a score of 13 out of 16), followed by Israel, Turkey, Egypt, the UAE, and Iran. Both Israel and Tunisia scored 36 out of 40 on the indicator of "political rights," followed by Turkey, Egypt, the UAE, and Iran. On the indicator of "level of violent crime," the UAE led (with the least level of violent crime) with a score of 1 out of 5 (1 = low; 5 = high), followed by Iran, Israel, Tunisia, Turkey, and Egypt (Fig. 5.12). It is to be noted that the wealthiest MENA countries (with high GDP per capita) such as the Emirates and Israel perform within the expected range on the indicator of "corruption" scoring, respectively, 66 and 64 out of 100 (0 = high; 100 = low), followed by Tunisia (with a grade or 41), Turkey (with a grade of 41), and Egypt (with a grade of 34). Iran, however, scored relatively high on the indicator of "corruption" with a grade of 29 (Table 5.5 and Fig. 5.12).

5.5 Information Communication Technology in the Middle East and North Africa Region: A Comparative Analysis

Access to communication technology has given rise to a quintessential shift in information-seeking behavior and is rapidly transforming the production, distribution, and consumption of knowledge and information in many parts of the world (el-Aswad 2014a). Knowledge-based economy is contingent on "information, technology and learning" (Organization for Economic Co-operation and Development (1996: 3). Use of communication technologies such as the Internet, mobile phones, Facebook, Twitter, and YouTube have had significant impact on socioeconomic activities and civil society in MENA countries (el-Aswad 2014b, c). Internet penetration in the MENA region reached 64.5% of the population in 2017 compared to the worldwide average of 54.5% (Internet World Stats 2017, 2018a). Three MENA countries are included in the top 20 nations of Internet users worldwide as of the year 2017: Iran (ranked 17), Turkey (ranked 18), and Egypt (ranked 20) (Internet World Stats 2018b).

Every country has the potential for achieving a high quality of life and well-being by maximizing the use of technology. However, the importance of ICTs to a government's vision varies among MENA countries. According to the Networked Readiness Index 2015, along this parameter, the UAE ranked first globally, followed by Israel (26), Turkey (73), Tunisia (90), Iran (91), and Egypt (112). The same pattern recurred concerning the driver of "government success in ICT promotion" such that the UAE ranked first globally, followed by Israel (22), Turkey (73), Tunisia (83), Iran (90), and Egypt (99). On the indicator of the "impact of ICTs on access to basic services," the UAE ranked fourth globally, followed by Israel (21), Turkey (46), Iran (91), Egypt (108), and Tunisia (110) (Table 5.4).

Information technology input indicators in Egypt include mobile phone subscriptions that reached 111 subscribers per 100 people and Internet users that reached 30 million or 32.6% of the population in 2015 compared to 438,208 users or 0.6% of the population in 2000 (Internet Live Stats 2016). As the population of young people in the MENA region has increased, communication technologies have expanded. In Iran, mobile phone subscriptions were recorded at 109 per 100 people in 2015, whereas Internet users reached more than 36 million, comprising 46% of the population compared to 615,165 users or 0.9% of the population in 2000. With the lifting of economic sanctions in 2016, Iran has become one of the most interesting and all-embracing telecom markets in the MENA countries, with more than 39 million Internet users comprising 48.9% of the population (Internet Live Stats 2016) (Fig. 5.13).

Mobile phone subscriptions in Israel reached 133.5 subscribers per 100 people (United Nations Development Programme 2016a), whereas Internet users increased from 1,255,289 or 20.9% of the population in 2000 to more than 5 million users or 72.2% of the population in 2015 (Internet Live Stats 2016). In Tunisia, mobile phone subscriptions numbered 129.9 per 100 people, whereas Internet users reached more than 5 million or 47.5% of the population compared to 266,800 users or 2.8% of the population in 2000 (Internet Live Stats 2016). According to the United Nations Development Programme (2016a), mobile phone subscriptions in Turkey were 102 per 100 people in 2015, whereas Internet users reached more than 43 million, or 53.7% of the population in 2015 (United Nations Development Programme 2016a) compared to 2,378,896 users or 0.9% of the population in 2000 (Internet Live Stats 2016). Internet users in the UAE increased from 26.6% of the population in 2000 to 91.2% by 2015 (see Fig. 4.1). Mobile phone subscriptions in the same year were

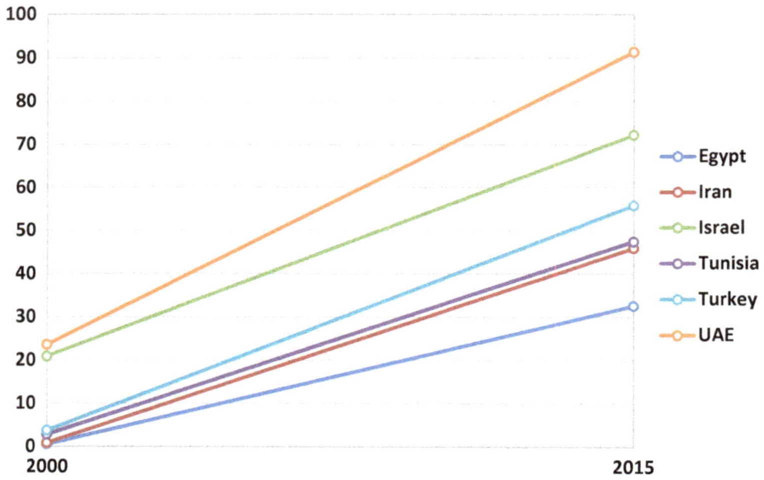

Fig. 5.13 Internet users in the Middle East and North Africa region, 2000–2015 (Data from Internet Live Stats 2016)

187.3 per 100 people (United Nations Development Programme 2016a). The UAE has embraced e-government and smart-government initiatives, with mobile Internet as part of their future progress (The National 2013).

Mobile phones and the Internet are used in these countries not only for information and educational purposes, but also for entertainment and online contacts and for exchanges of personal and social views. The one-way communication of radio, television, and print media provide information to an audience but cannot solicit immediate feedback. On the contrary, the two-way communications of the Internet and cyber network encourage social and cultural engagement and allow for mutual feedback (el-Aswad 2014a, b).

5.6 Social Policies

In addition to public policies and recommendations provided for each of the selected MENA countries, this section proposes key broad policy options targeting the MENA region as a whole to help policy makers find better ways to improve the level and distribution of well-being outcomes.

The social-public policy is expected to improve not only public-sector services but also the relationship between people and the government (Silva et at. 2012; Yaghi and Al-Jenaibi 2018). One of the most critical policies that needs to be implemented is to decentralize government institutions to increase life satisfaction and help people become happy. It is also urgent to set policies aimed at reducing the rapid population growth rates in most of the MENA countries, particularly Egypt, Iran, and Turkey. For instance, in 2017, the Egyptian Prime Minister warned that unprecedented population growth is the biggest challenge to the country (Ahramonline 2017).

More efficient policies are needed to improve health-related well-being by increasing budgets for public health provisions to support hospitals, clinics, and health insurance systems and to augment the income or salaries of doctors, nurses, and other medical professionals, particularly in medium- and low-income states. More effective policies are required to protect people with special needs, the poor, and the vulnerable, including the elderly and the refugees.

The role of education as a driver to well-being should be examined and enhanced. It is necessary to improve the quality of education at all levels, including preprimary to higher education, by increasing funding, updating curricula, boosting administrative systems, recruiting and training highly qualified instructors, and building reliable educational facilities.

Technology and innovation, the highest manifestation of human creativity, are among the most powerful input indicators impacting the progress of quality of life and well-being (Selian and McKnight 2017). The application of advanced technology and innovation in all domains of life must be a priority for public policies in all of the MENA states.

Specific institutions of Islamic care and counseling (public and private) have created Web sites and online services broadly reaching clients and receivers in the MENA region. These Web sites allow people comprising a large number of online consumers in the MENA countries to partake freely in discussing certain aspects of health (el-Aswad 2017).

Culture is a powerful driver for the development and well-being of people. Culture can be defined as "the set of distinctive spiritual, material, intellectual and emotional features of a society or a social group" (United Nations Research Institute for Social Development 2013: 12). One of the significant roles of culture is represented in its contribution to education, health, and economy. Cultural heritage, cultural art, cultural creative industries, sustainable cultural tourism, and cultural infrastructure can serve as strategic mechanisms for revenue generation, particularly in developing countries, given their rich cultural heritage and substantial labor force (UNESCO 2012; World Bank 2001, 2015).

Comprehensive social-public policy plans are needed to activate civil society by launching national and regional programs that motivate people, particularly the youth and women, to actively engage and participate in public life and civic initiatives. It is important for policy makers to support dynamic and strong private, informal sectors as well as to encourage stakeholders to participate in policy processes that can reduce unemployment and create jobs and opportunities for people, particularly the youth (male and female) in the MENA region. Policy makers and governments of the region must provide well designed policy issues to ensure employment opportunities for the unemployed, particularly among the young who represent about 30% of the total population (Keulertz et al. 2016).

Regional partnerships and collaboration in the domains of public goods and sectors such as health, education, security, and trade are necessary for improving the quality of life of those in the MENA countries. More efforts are needed to support public and political policies that provide initiatives to solve geopolitical conflicts and political instability across the MENA region especially for those experiencing instability and strife.

Generally, MENA states should move beyond short-term plans that focus on temporary issues such as food and fuel subsidies, to embrace long-term policies focusing on improving human capital as well as on eliminating inequalities in well-being within and across the different MENA countries. Additionally, MENA governments should use well-being research outcomes to formulate strategic initiatives for the development of cultural policies to sustain and spend on cultural endeavors, including heritage and art, as key drivers toward improving quality of life in the region.

5.7 Conclusion

This chapter has provided a background of the key drivers of well-being and policy issues that have shaped the quality of life in the MENA region with particular focus on the domains of health, education, economy, and technology within the identified countries of Egypt, Iran, Israel, Tunisia, Turkey, and the UAE.

This study has highlighted that both the governments and the grassroot populations of the MENA states work diligently to improve their standards of living. There has been progressive and ongoing development in the domains of health, education, economy, and technology that has impacted positively on the overall quality of life of the MENA region.

The chapter has shown that examination of the drivers and input indicator outcomes of well-being can guide the policy decisions of governments and actors working within a broad range of economic, health, and educational institutions.

Key priorities for the MENA region continue to be emboldening employment and making health services, education, and economies more all-encompassing to meet the population's demands for a higher quality of life.

References

Ahmed, M. (2016). MENA's private education sector: A burgeoning market. *Newsweek*. Retrieved from http://newsweekme.com/menas-private-education-sector-burgeoning-market/.

Ahramonline. (2017). *Unprecedented population growth' is Egypt's biggest challenge, PM Ismail tells House*. Retrieved from http://english.ahram.org.eg/NewsContent/1/64/278149/Egypt/Politics-/Unprecedented-population-growth-is-Egypts-biggest-.aspx.

Al Masah Capital. (2016). *MENA Yearbook*. Dubai, UAE: Al Masah Capital Management Limited. Retrieved from http://www.almasahcapital.com/images/reports/report_144.pdf.

Al Masah Capital. (2018). *MENA Yearbook*. Dubai, UAE: Al Masah Capital Management Limited.

Arab Barometer (2011). *Arab Republic of Egypt*. Retrieved from http://www.arabbarometer.org/content/arab-barometer-ii-egypt.

Arab Barometer. (2013). *Online data analysis: Trust, civil society institutions*. Retrieved from http://www.arabbarometer.org/content/online-data-analysis.

Arabian Business. (2016). *UAE's $13.3bn budget for 2017 to focus on education, healthcare.* Retrieved from http://www.arabianbusiness.com/uae-s-13-3bn-budget-for-2017-focus-on-education-healthcare-657122.html.

Arani, A., Kakai, L., Taghavi, T. (2015). Privatization of education in the Islamic Republic of Iran: One step forward, one step back. *Cogent Education, 2*(1), 1029709. Retrieved from https://www.tandfonline.com/doi/full/10.1080/2331186X.2015.1029709, https://doi.org/10.1080/2331186x.2015.1029709.

Bertelsmann Stiftung, B. T. I. (2016). *United Arab Emirates Country Report*. Gütersloh, Germany: Bertelsmann Stiftung. Retrieved from https://www.bti-project.org/fileadmin/files/BTI/Downloads/Reports/2016/pdf/BTI_2016_United_Arab_Emirates.pdf.

Bremer, J. (2015). Challenges to governance reform and accountability in Egypt. In A. Dawoody (Ed.), *Public administration and policy in the Middle East* (pp. 82–101). New York: Springer.

Central Intelligence Agency. (2018). *The world factbook*. Washington, DC: Central Intelligence Agency. Retrieved from https://www.cia.gov/library/publications/the-world-factbook/fields/2103.html.

Cochran, J. (2017). Israel: Divided by religion and education. *Digest of the Middle East Studies, 26*(1), 32–55.

Daily Sabah. (2016). *Health: Smoking ban in Turkey, 7 years later, turns tide on prevalent habit.* Retrieved from https://www.dailysabah.com/health/2016/07/19/smoking-ban-in-turkey-7-years-later-turns-tide-on-prevalent-habit.

Deloitte. (2016). 2016 *Global health care outlook: Regional and country perspectives.* Retrieved from https://www2.deloitte.com/content/dam/Deloitte/global/Documents/Life-Sciences-Health-Care/gx-lshc-2016-health-care-outlook-regional.pdf.

Dubai Health Authority (2018). [Organization Web site]. Retrieved from https://www.dha.gov.ae/en/pages/dhahome.aspx.

Dubai International Academic City. (2018). Retrieved from http://www.diacedu.ae.

Dubai Knowledge Village. (2018). Retrieved from http://www.dkp.ae.

Eickelman, D. (1992). The re-imagination of the Middle East: Political and academic frontiers. *Middle East Studies Association Bulletin, 26*(1), 3–12.

Eickelman, D., & Piscatori, J. (1996). *Muslim Politics*. Princeton, NJ: Princeton University Press.

Eickelman, D. (2008). Gender and religion in the public and private sphere. In K. Ohtsuka & D. F. Eickelman (Eds.), *Crossing boundaries: Gender and the public, and the private in contemporary Muslim societies* (pp. 135–150). Tokyo: Research Institute for Languages and Cultures of Asia and Africa.

el-Aswad, el-S. (2010). The perceptibility of the invisible cosmology: Religious rituals and embodied spirituality among the Bahraini Shi'a. *Anthropology of the Middle East, 5*(2), 59–76.

el-Aswad, el-S. (2012). *Muslim worldviews and everyday lives*. Lanham, MD: AltaMira Press, Rowman & Littlefield Publisher.

el-Aswad, el-S. (2014a). E-folklore and cyber-communication among Emirati youth. *International Journal of Intangible Heritage, 9*, 49–62.

el-Aswad, el-S. (2014b). Communication. In K. Harvey (Ed.), *Encyclopedia of social media and politics* (Vol. 1, pp. 304–308). Thousand Oaks, CA: Sage.

el-Aswad, el-S. (2014c). Social worlds. In K. Harvey (Ed.), *Encyclopedia of social media and politics* (Vol. 2, pp. 1190–1192). Thousand Oaks, CA: Sage.

el-Aswad, el-S. (2015). From traditional charity to global philanthropy: Dynamics of the spirit of giving and volunteerism in the United Arab Emirates. *Horizons in Humanities and Social Sciences: An International Refereed Journal, 1*(1), 1–21.

el-Aswad, el-S. (2017). Islamic care and counseling. In D. A. Leeming, (Ed.), *Encyclopaedia of psychology and religion* (pp. 1–14). Berlin/Heidelberg: Springer Verlag. https://doi.org/10.1007/978-3-642-27771-9_200074-1.

El-Megharbel, N. (2015). *Sustainable development strategy of Egypt: Egypt's vision 2030 and planning reform.* Retrieved from https://sustainabledevelopment.un.org/content/documents/15262El-Megharbell,%20Egypt%20NSDS%2020150527.pdf.

Financing Global Health. (2016). *Financing global health 2016: Development assistance, public and private health spending for the pursuit of universal health coverage.* Seattle, WA: Institute for Health Metrics and Evaluation. Retrieved from http://www.healthdata.org/sites/default/files/files/policy_report/fgh/2017/ihme_fgh2016_technical-report.pdf.

Gabbay, Y. (2016, February 18). Israel at an economic-policy crossroads. *Haaretz*. Retrieved from https://www.haaretz.com/israel-news/business/.premium-israel-at-an-economic-crossroads-1.5405807.

Gal, J., & Madhala, S. (2017). *Developments in Israeli social welfare policy*. Jerusalem: Taub Center for Social Policy Studies in Israel. Retrieved from http://taubcenter.org.il/wp-content/files_mf/developmentsinsocialwelfarepolicy.pdf.

Gomaa, A., et al. (2017). Hepatitis C infection in Egypt: Prevalence, impact and management strategies. *Hepatic Medicine: Evidence and Research, 9,* 17–25. https://doi.org/10.2147/HMER.S113681.

Goudarzi, S., et al. (2011). Improvement in health indicators of Islamic Republic of Iran in the years 2004 and 2008. *Irananian Red Crescent Medical Journal, 13*(8), 574–577.

Gürbüz, Ş. M. (2017). Important steps taken in Turkey's social policy, but the best is yet to come. *Daily Sabah: Politics*. Retrieved from https://www.dailysabah.com/politics/2017/06/25/important-steps-taken-in-turkeys-social-policy-but-the-best-is-yet-to-come.

Halm, H. (2007). *The Shi'ates: A Short History* (A. Brown, Trans.). Princeton, NJ: Markus Wiener Publishers.

Hamann, T., & Rosen, L. (2011). What makes the anthropology of educational policy implementation "anthropological"? In B. Levinson & M. Pollock (Eds.), *A companion to the anthropology of education* (pp. 461–477). New York: Wiley Blackwell.

Heyneman, S. P. (1997). The quality of education in the Middle East and North Africa (MENA). *International Journal of Educational Development, 17*(4), 449–466.

Health Authority Abu Dhabi (2018). [Web site]. Retrieved from https://www.haad.ae/haad/.

Huppert, F. A., & Cooper, C. L. (2014). *Interventions and policies to enhance wellbeing: A complete reference guide* (Vol. VI). Chichester, West Sussex: Wiley.

International Labor Organization. (2017). *Tunisia*. Retrieved from http://www.ilo.org/dyn/normlex/en/f?p=NORMLEXPUB:11110:0::NO::P11110_COUNTRY_ID:102986.

Internet Live Stats. (2016). *Internet users by country*. Retrieved from http://www.internetlivestats.com/internet-users-by-country/.

Internet World Stats. (2017). *Iran*. Retrieved from http://www.internetworldstats.com/me/ir.htm.

Internet World Stats. (2018a). *Internet usage in the Middle East*. Retrieved from https://www.internetworldstats.com/stats5.htm.

Internet World Stats. (2018b). *Top 20 countries with the highest number of Internet users* 2017. Retrieved from https://www.internetworldstats.com/top20.htm.

Jawad, R. (2008). *Social policy in the Middle East. Policy World (Spring: 8–12)*. Retrieved from http://www.social-policy.org.uk/wordpress/wp-content/uploads/2014/05/PolicyWorld_Spr08.pdf.

Jawad, R. (2015). *Social protection and social policy systems in the MENA region: Emerging trends*. New York: United Nations Department of Economic and Social Affairs.

Karshenas, M, & Moghadam, V. M. (2009). Bringing social policy back in: A look at the Middle East and North Africa. *International Journal of Social Welfare, 18*(s1), S52–S61.

Keulertz, M. et al. (2016). *Material factors for the MENA Region: Data sources, trends and drivers. Middle East and North Africa Regional Architecture*. Retrieved from https://www.cidob.org/content/download/65695/2014964/version/12/file/MENARA%20Concep%20paper%203_16.pdf.

Keyes, C. L. (1998). Social well-being. *Social Psychology Quarterly, 61*(2), 121–140.

Khaleej Times. (2018). *One-month bonus for all government staff on Zayed centenary*. Retrieved from https://www.khaleejtimes.com/news/government/sheikh-khalifa-orders-salary-bonus-to-all-government-employees.

Koornneef, E. et al. (2017). Progress and outcomes of health systems reform in the United Arab Emirates: A systematic review. *BMC Health Services Research, 17*, 672. https://doi.org/10.1186/

s12913-017-2597-1. Retrieved from https://bmchealthservres.biomedcentral.com/track/pdf/10.1186/s12913-017-2597-1?site=bmchealthservres.biomedcentral.com.

Lammy, D, & Tyler, B. C. (2014). *Wellbeing in four policy areas: Report by the all-party parliamentary group on wellbeing economics*. Retrieved from http://b.3cdn.net/nefoundation/ccdf9782b6d8700f7c_lcm6i2ed7.pdf.

Lankarani, K., et al. (2013). Health in the Islamic Republic of Iran, challenges and progresses. *Medical Journal of the Islam Republic of Iran, 27*(1), 42–49.

Layard, R. (2005). *Happiness: Lessons from a new science*. London: Penguin Books.

Leavy, A. (2010). *The failure of educational policy in Israel: Politics versus bureaucracy* (Unpublished thesis). University of Pennsylvania. Retrieved from https://repository.upenn.edu/cgi/viewcontent.cgi?article=1136&context=curej.

Louër, L. (2008). *Transnational Shia politics: Religious and political networks in the Gulf*. New York: Columbia University Press.

Michalos, A. C. (2007). *Education, happiness and wellbeing*. Paper written for the International Conference on 'Is happiness measurable and what do those measures mean for public policy?', Rome, 2–3 April 2007, University of Rome. Retrieved from http://search.oecd.org/site/worldforum06/38303200.pdf.

Ministry of Education, Islamic Republic of Iran. (2011). *Fundamental reform document of education (FRDE) in the Islamic Republic of Iran*. Retrieved from http://www.dres.ir/safeschool/Downloads/FRDE.pdf.

Ministry of Education, Israel. (2018). [Web site]. Retrieved from http://edu.gov.il/owlHeb/AboutUs/FreedomOfInformation/Pages/english.aspx.

Ministry of Education, Republic of Tunisia (2018). [Web site]. [Arabic]. Retrieved from http://www.education.gov.tn/index.php?id=397&lan=3#?.

Ministry of Health and Population, Egypt. (2018). [Web site]. [Arabic]. Retrieved from http://www.mohp.gov.eg.

Ministry of Health of Turkey. (2012). *Strategic plan* 2013–2017. Retrieved from https://sgb.saglik.gov.tr/Dkmanlar/Strategic%20Plan%202013-2017.pdf.

Nuseibeh, R. A. (2016). *Political conflict and exclusion in Jerusalem: The provision of education and social services*. London: Routledge.

Organization for Economic Co-operation and Development. (1996). *The knowledge-based economy*. Paris: Organization for Economic Co-operation and Development. Retrieved from https://www.oecd.org/sti/sci-tech/1913021.pdf.

Organization for Economic Cooperation and Development. (2013). *Education policy outlook: Turkey*. Retrieved from http://www.oecd.org/education/EDUCATION%20POLICY%20OUTLOOK%20TURKEY_EN.pdf.

Organization for Economic Cooperation and Development. (2015a). *Measuring and assessing well-being in Israel*. Paris: OECD Publishing. Retrieved from http://mof.gov.il/chiefecon/internationalconnections/oecd/oecd_wellbeingreport.pdf.

Organization for Economic Cooperation and Development. (2015b). *Tunisia: A reform agenda to support competitiveness and inclusive growth*. Better Policies Series: Tunisia. Retrieved from https://www.oecd.org/economy/Tunisia-a-reform-agenda-to-support-competitiveness-and-inclusive-growth.pdf.

Organization for Economic Cooperation and Development. (2016a). *Education policy outlook: Israel*. Retrieved from http://www.oecd.org/education/Education-Policy-Outlook-Country-Profile-Israel.pdf.

Organization for Economic Cooperation and Development. (2016b). *Middle East and North Africa*. Retrieved from http://www.oecd.org/mena/Active_with_MENA_EN.pdf.

Oxford Business Group. (2016). *Health and education in Tunisia*. Retrieved from https://oxfordbusinessgroup.com/tunisia-2016/health-education.

Oxford Business Group. (2018). *Egypt: Education. Egypt increases spending on education and improves quality and access*. Retrieved from https://oxfordbusinessgroup.com/overview/focus-point-increase-spending-should-support-aim-improving-quality-well-access.

Parsa, P. et al. (2012). Effect of prenatal health care on pregnancy outcomes in Hamadan, Iran. *Journal of Community Medicine and Health Education, 2*, 114. https://doi.org/10.4172/2161-0711.1000114. Retrieved from https://www.omicsonline.org/effect-of-prenatal-health-care-on-pregnancy-outcomes-in-hamadan-iran-2161-0711.1000114.php?aid=3545.

Rosen, B., et al. (2015). Health system review. *Health Systems in Transition, 17*(6), 1–212.

Republic of Turkey. (2014). *Tenth development plan* (2014–2018). Retrieved from http://www.mod.gov.tr/Lists/RecentPublications/Attachments/75/The%20Tenth%20Development%20Plan%20(2014–2018).pdf.

Sachs, J. (2005). *The end of poverty: How we can make it happen in our lifetime*. London: Penguin Books.

Saeidi, A. A. (2009). Iranian Para-governmental Organizations (bonyads). *Middle East Institute.* Retrieved from http://www.mei.edu/content/iranian-para-governmental-organizations-bonyads.

Sakurai, K. (2017). Western and Islamic models of higher education in Saudi Arabia and Iran. In D. F. Eickelman & R. M. Abusharaf (Eds.), *Higher education investment in the Arab States of the Gulf: Strategies for excellence and diversity* (pp. 23–41). Berlin: Gerlach Press.

Selian, A. N., & McKnight, L. (2017). The role of technology in the history of well-being: Transformative market phenomena over time. In R. J. Estes & M. J. Sirgy (Eds.), *The pursuit of human well-being: The untold global history* (pp. 639–687). Dordrecht, NL: Springer.

Silva, J., Levin, V., & Morgand, M. (2012). *The way forward for social safety nets in the Middle East and North Africa*. Washington DC: World Bank.

Sirgy, M. J., Estes, R. J., & Selian, A. N. (2017). How we measure well-being: The data behind the history of well-being. In R. J. Estes & M. J. Sirgy (Eds.), *The pursuit of human well-being: The untold global history* (pp. 135–160). Dordrecht, NL: Springer.

Social Progress Index. (2017). Retrieved from http://www.socialprogressimperative.org and http://www.socialprogressindex.com/assets/downloads/resources/en/English-2017-Social-Progress-Index-Findings-Report_embargo-d-until-June-21-2017.pdf.

Sputnik news. (2018). *Iran moves to lessen Guard presence in economy*. Retrieved from https://sputniknews.com/business/201801221060947398-iran-revolutionary-guard-economy/.

Statista-Statistics Portal. (2017). *Internet user penetration in Egypt from 2013 to 2019*. Retrieved from https://www.statista.com/statistics/484939/internet-user-reach-egypt/.

Sustainable Governance Indicators. (2016). *Israel: Social policies*. Retrieved from http://www.sgi-network.org/2016/Israel/Social_Policies.

The National. (2013). *UAE has third most internet users in the Middle East*. Retrieved from https://www.thenational.ae/business/uae-has-third-most-internet-users-in-the-middle-east-1.447311.

The National. (2017). *UAE parents are the second highest education spenders globally*. Retrieved from https://www.thenational.ae/business/money/uae-parents-are-the-second-highest-education-spenders-globally-1.663348.

The National. (2018). *President orders payment of one month salary to all Government employees*. Retrieved from https://www.thenational.ae/uae/president-orders-payment-of-one-month-salary-to-all-government-employees-1.727511.

UNESCO. (2012). *Culture: A driver and an enabler of sustainable development: Thematic Think Piece. UN System Task Team on the Post-2015 UN Development Agenda*. Retrieved from http://www.un.org/millenniumgoals/pdf/Think%20Pieces/2_culture.pdf.

UNESCO. (2017). Country strategy for the Islamic Republic of Iran 2017–2021. Retrieved from http://unesdoc.unesco.org/images/0026/002602/260299e.pdf.

UNESCO. (2018a). *Egypt*. Retrieved from http://uis.unesco.org/en/country/EG.

UNESCO. (2018b). *Iran*. Retrieved from http://uis.unesco.org/en/country/ir.

UNESCO. (2018c). *Israel*. Retrieved from http://uis.unesco.org/en/country/il.

UNESCO. (2018d). *Tunisia*. Retrieved from http://uis.unesco.org/en/country/tn.

UNESCO. (2018e). *Turkey*. Retrieved from http://uis.unesco.org/en/country/tr.

UNESCO. (2018f). *United Arab Emirates*. Retrieved from http://uis.unesco.org/en/country/ae.

UNICEF. (2015a). *Middle East and North Africa out of school children initiative. Regional report on out-of-school children.* Retrieved from http://unesdoc.unesco.org/images/0023/002326/232689e.pdf.

UNICEF. (2015b). *Middle East and North Africa out of school children initiative. Tunisia: Country report on out-of-school children.* Retrieved from http://www.oosci-mena.org/uploads/1/wysiwyg/summary/150310_Tunisia_summary_English_Preview.pdf.

UNICEF. (2016a). *Annual report 2015.* Retrieved from https://www.unicef.org/publications/files/UNICEF_Annual_Report_2015_En.pdf.

UNICEF. (2016b). *UNICEF Annual Report 2016: Tunisia.* Retrieved from https://www.unicef.org/about/annualreport/files/Tunisia_2016_COAR.pdf.

UNICEF. (2017). *UNICEF Annual Report 2017: Egypt.* Retrieved from https://www.unicef.org/about/annualreport/files/Egypt_2017_COAR.pdf.

UNICEF-OOSCI. (2018). *Middle East and North Africa out-of-school children initiative.* Retrieved from http://www.oosci-mena.org/.

United Arab Emirates. (2014). *UAE vision 2021 national agenda.* Retrieved from https://uaecabinet.ae/en/national-agenda and http://rwadubai.com/media/2578/uae-national-agenda.pdf.

United Arab Emirates Ministry of Education. (2018). *Ministry of education strategic* plan 2017–2021. Retrieved from https://www.moe.gov.ae/En/AboutTheMinistry/Pages/MinistryStrategy.aspx.

United Arab Emirates Ministry of Health and Prevention. (2018). *MOHAP strategy.* Retrieved from http://www.mohap.gov.ae/en/aboutus/Pages/Strategy.aspx.

United Nations Development Assistance Framework. (2013). *Egypt* 2013–2017. Retrieved from http://www.undp.org/content/dam/egypt/docs/LegalFramework/UNDAF%202013-2017.pdf.

United Nations Development Assistance Framework. (2015). *Islamic Republic of Iran* 2017–2021. Retrieved from https://www.unicef.org/about/execboard/files/Iran_UNDAF_2017-2021.pdf.

United Nations Development Programme. (2016a). *Human development index.* Retrieved from http://hdr.undp.org/en/indicators/137506.

United Nations Development Programme. (2016b). *Human development report 2016. Human development for everyone.* Retrieved from http://hdr.undp.org/sites/default/files/HDR2016_EN_Overview_Web.pdf.

United Nations High Commissioner for Refugees. (2016). *Global trends: Forced displacement in 2016.* Retrieved from www.unhcr.org/5943e8a34.pdf.

United Nations Research Institute for Social Development. (2013). *Social drivers of sustainable development.* Retrieved from http://www.unrisd.org/social-drivers-note.

University of California San Francisco Global Health Group. (2015). *Eliminating malaria in Iran.* Retrieved from https://globalhealthsciences.ucsf.edu/sites/globalhealthsciences.ucsf.edu/files/pub/iran2015-final.pdf.

Walker, T. (2012). *International study links higher teacher pay and teacher quality.* Retrieved from *neaToday*: http://neatoday.org/2012/01/04/international-study-links-higher-teacher-pay-and-teacher-quality/.

World Bank (2001). *Cultural heritage and development: A framework for action in the Middle East and North Africa.* Washington, DC: Orientations in Development series. Retrieved from https://openknowledge.worldbank.org/handle/10986/13908.

World Bank. (2008). *Health and the Islamic republic of Iran: Human development sector Middle East and North Africa.* Orientations in development series. Washington, DC: World Bank.

World Bank. (2015). *Our new strategy.* Retrieved from http://www.worldbank.org/en/region/mena/brief/our-new-strategy.

World Bank. (2016). *Tunisia moves to modernize its social protection and labor policies.* Retrieved from http://www.worldbank.org/en/news/feature/2016/05/20/tunisia-moves-to-modernize-its-social-protection.

World Bank. (2017a). *The world bank in Egypt.* Retrieved from http://www.worldbank.org/en/country/egypt/overview.

World Bank. (2017b). *Islamic Republic of Iran*. Retrieved from http://www.worldbank.org/en/country/iran/overview.

World Bank. (2017c). *United Arab Emirates*. Retrieved from https://data.worldbank.org/country/united-arab-emirates.

World Bank. (2018a). *Pregnant women receiving prenatal care (%)*. Retrieved from https://data.worldbank.org/indicator/SH.STA.ANVC.ZS?locations=IL-IR.

World Bank (2018b). *Government expenditure on education, total (% of GDP)*. Retrieved from https://data.worldbank.org/indicator/SE.XPD.TOTL.GD.ZS?locations=EG-IR-IL-TN.

World Bank. (2018c). *World bank provides US$500 million to Egypt for improving teaching and learning conditions in public schools*. Retrieved from http://www.worldbank.org/en/news/press-release/2018/04/13/world-bank-provides-us500-million-to-egypt-for-improving-teaching-and-learning-conditions-in-public-schools.

World Bank. (2018d). *Physicians (per 1000 people)*. Retrieved from https://data.worldbank.org/indicator/SH.MED.PHYS.ZS?locations=EG-IL-IR-TN-TR-AE.

World Data Atlas. (2018a). *Egypt: Private expenditure on health as a share of total health expenditure*. Retrieved from https://knoema.com/atlas/Egypt/topics/Health/Health-Expenditure/Private-expenditure-on-health-as-a-share-of-total-health-expenditure.

World Data Atlas. (2018b). *Iran: Social health insurance as a share of current health expenditure*. Retrieved from https://knoema.com/atlas/Iran/topics/Health/Health-Expenditure/Social-health-insurance-as-a-share-of-current-health-expenditure.

World Data Atlas. (2018c). *Tunisia: Social health insurance as a share of current health expenditure*. Retrieved from https://knoema.com/atlas/Tunisia/topics/Health/Health-Expenditure/Social-health-insurance-as-a-share-of-current-health-expenditure.

World Food Programme. (2018). *Draft Tunisia country strategic plan* (2018–2022). Retrieved from https://docs.wfp.org/api/documents/40c35cf3-4055-4588-9c89-e3e59ac6a483/download/.

World Economic Forum. (2016). *The global information technology report 2016: Innovating in the digital economy*. Geneva: World Economic Forum. Retrieved from http://www3.weforum.org/docs/GITR2016/WEF_GITR_Full_Report.pdf.

World Economic Forum. (2017). *Global competitiveness report 2016–17*. Geneva: World Economic Forum. Retrieved from http://www3.weforum.org/docs/GCR2016-2017/05FullReport/TheGlobalCompetitivenessReport2016-2017_FINAL.pdf.

World Health Organization. (2016). *United Arab Emirates: Diabetes country profiles, 2016*. Retrieved from http://www.who.int/diabetes/country-profiles/are_en.pdf.

World Health Organization. (2017). *World health statistics 2017: Monitoring health for the SDGs, Sustainable development goals*. Retrieved from http://apps.who.int/iris/bitstream/10665/255336/1/9789241565486-eng.pdf?ua=1.

World Health Organization. (2018). *Global health observatory (GHO) data: Life expectancy*. Retrieved from http://www.who.int/gho/mortality_burden_disease/life_tables/situation_trends_text/en/.

Yaghi, A., & Al-Jenaibi, B. (2018). Happiness, morality, rationality, and challenges in implementing smart government policy. *Public Integrity, 20*(3), 284–299. https://doi.org/10.1080/10999922.2017.1364947.

Yousef, T. M. (2004). Development, growth and policy reform in the Middle East and North Africa since 1950. *Journal of Economic Perspectives, 18*(3), 91–116.

Chapter 6
Conclusion

Abstract This chapter provides a concise yet essential conclusion highlighting the main findings of the monograph pertaining to quality of life and policy issues among Middle East and North African countries. These findings are addressed by focusing on central points with specific reference to cross-cultural inquiry, historical perspective, progression and regression of quality of life and well-being, and effectiveness of social policy.

Keywords Cross-cultural approach · Quality of life · Well-being · Social policy

6.1 Introduction

This book has dealt with quality of life and policy issues among 21 countries of the Middle East and North African (MENA) region, which until now have not been examined cross-culturally in sufficient depth. This research has tackled a critical topic encompassing such interrelated and complicated themes as development, quality of life, drivers of well-being, and policy issues in the MENA region. Put differently, this book, focusing on both objective and subjective dimensions of well-being, has attempted to portray a single holistic picture of quality of life and well-being among the MENA countries despite the vast diversity of historical, political, and economic features and events that they have experienced as well as the various cultural characteristics they possess.

6.1.1 Cross-Cultural and Historical Perspectives

In addition to scholarly work addressing sociological and historical issues, this research has used cross-cultural perspectives using information and global measures collected from world's largest data collection and reporting agencies. This book has provided a background of the key drivers of well-being and policy issues that have

el-S. el-Aswad, *The Quality of Life and Policy Issues among the Middle East and North African Countries*, Human Well-Being Research and Policy Making,
https://doi.org/10.1007/978-3-030-00326-5_6

shaped the quality of life in the MENA region. It has applied multiple objective and subjective indicators to assess the multifaceted dimensions of well-being including health, education, economy, work force, communication technology, human rights, happiness, religious freedom, security, political stability, tolerance, political terror, corruption, and freedom of expression, to mention a few. Cross-culturally, examples of certain dimensions of well-being prevailing in the MENA countries have been provided to illustrate the similarities and differences between them. Further, this book presents a comparative analysis focusing on indicators of equity and inequality in differing domains of human development and well-or ill-being. For example, the level of income inequality between men and women is low in some countries such as Israel, Turkey, the United Arab Emirates (UAE), and Egypt, compared to other countries such Iran and Tunisia, in which the disparity is very high. But, with women becoming increasingly more educated than in the past and more involved in activities outside the household, women's social and economic roles have become more visible. Policy issues that address inequalities in well-being within and across different MENA countries will have a positive impact on reducing regional inequalities.

This monograph has provided a broad account of the region's core geographic, demographic, and political features as well as of the inclusive human development, particularly in the domains of economy, health, education, technology, and political stability. This study has traced in broad terms the achievements, challenges, and overall human development trajectory experienced by people in the MENA region from ancient times to the present. No one specific pattern of quality of life or well-being holds for the entire Middle East. The MENA region is characterized by a rich historical past, which has had major sociocultural, religious, and political impacts regionally and globally. Historical events have played a significant role in shaping certain dimensions of well-being in the MENA region. This monograph has shown that the quality of life and well-being of the MENA people have traversed successive stages of progression and regression, sparked by exterior and interior drivers and factors, through various periods of ancient, medieval, and modern history.

The impact of culture on the MENA region's well-being and development of public policies is significant. The MENA region is rich with an extraordinary cultural heritage, both secular and religious, of eminent importance for each country and for humankind at large. Along with its enormous intangible heritage, the region is home to 48 world heritage sites identified and maintained by UNESCO (World Bank 2001).

It is worth pointing out that cultural and creative industries represent one of the most rapidly expanding sectors in the global economy with a growth rate of 17.6% in the Middle East, 13.9% in Africa, 11.9% in South America, 9.7% in Asia, 6.9% in Oceania, and 4.3% in North and Central America. Promoting cultural sectors requires limited capital investment and can have a direct impact on vulnerable populations, including women. Presently, many countries use cultural heritage and cultural events and institutions to improve their image and attract visitors and investments (UNESCO 2012). What is needed is to integrate traditional knowledge and other cultural elements into reasonable policies that have as their goal the improvement of the quality of life and well-being of the region's steadily increasing population.

6.1.2 Quality of Life and Well-Being

This monograph has identified important indicators and measurements of progress in people's economic, health, and educational development as a whole. It has also investigated the systems of social and public policies implemented in the MENA region impacting economic, health, and educational well-being.

This inquiry has extensively assessed the progress MENA countries have made over the past 25 years (1990–2015) in various aspects of quality of life and well-being. Despite the variations in quality of life across the MENA region, there is a common pattern of well-being related mainly to the progress made in the multiple dimensions of people's lives. The MENA region has been and continues to be one of the world's most swiftly developing regions. People in the region are better off than they were in 1990. In other words, this research has pointed out that MENA countries have made significant progress in almost all domains of well-being, despite the disparities and differences in the outcomes between the countries.

Progress is described in improved health care, longer life expectancy, longer years of schooling, increased rates of literacy, partial economic growth, and effective use of communication technology. For example, according to the 2015 Human Development Index (United Nations Development Programme 2016), six MENA countries (Bahrain, Israel, Kuwait, Qatar, Saudi Arabia, and the UAE) were included in the list of 51 countries ranked very high in human development. Eight MENA countries were among the 53 countries (including three of the selected countries) that ranked high. Four MENA countries were among the 41 countries (including one of the selected counties) that ranked medium. Three MENA countries were among the 53 countries that ranked low. In addition, three of the selected MENA countries performed very well in the Global Competitiveness Index conducted by the World Economic Forum in 2016–2017. The UAE, with a global rank of 16 (out of 138 countries) has led the MENA countries, followed by Israel (24) and Turkey (55) (World Economic Forum 2017). Further, utilization of communication technologies such as the Internet, mobile phones, Facebook, Twitter, and YouTube has had a significant impact on socioeconomic activities and civil society in MENA countries.

Although the MENA region has performed better than non-MENA countries, particularly in the areas of economic liberalization, such as size of the market and monetary policy, it is lagging in other areas, such as trade strategies, governmental involvement in the economy, foreign direct investment, and wage and price flexibility (Looney 2004). Besides, certain dimensions of well-being are lagging behind due to socioeconomic and political disparities and gender inequality. The uneven distribution of social, health, economic, and educational benefits has a negative impact on both quality of life and social policy in the MENA states. Overall, rates of unemployment of women are disproportionately high and women's participation in the labor force and political life is still small across the region.

Despite the quantitative development of education in terms of length of time in school and large enrollments of students, the quality of education in the MENA region is lagging behind. Furthermore, the demographic features of the region present another challenge, generating socioeconomic and political problems that need robust solutions. More than 29% of the population of the Middle East is between the ages of 15 and 29. The rapid increase in the number of young people, especially in the of 20–24 years old, aggravates the problem of unemployment. It is imperative to set policies designed to reduce the rapid population growth rates in most of the MENA countries, but most specifically in Egypt, Iran, and Turkey.

Inequality, lack of democracy, and inflexible government systems, seriously felt amid profound political disruptions in most of the MENA countries, generate a vicious circle leading to failure of social-public policy that, in turn, results in poor quality of life, the rise of extremism and terrorism, and social-political instability. In brief, indicators of freedom of expression, religious tolerance, and happiness are still low in most MENA countries. For instance, the level of happiness in Iran and Tunisia has shown a continuous deterioration in both global score and rank.

Results clearly show that differences in well-being among the countries being studied are not necessarily in line with those based on their GDP level per capita. For instance, as shown in the study, countries with the same level of GDP per capita have different human development outcomes in the domains of health, education, social support, happiness, and life satisfaction. These differences are most likely related to ideological, political, and cultural orientations as well as to corrupt governmental management.

6.1.3 Social Policy: Governmental and Non-governmental Agencies

Social policy is a profoundly political process of sociocultural production involved in and formed by social actors in different locations that exert remarkable amounts of influence. The provision of good public services and trust in national, regional, and global public institutions such as governments, police forces, and legal systems, bring about high levels of well-being and life satisfaction. The shortage of these attributes results in ill-being, depleted states of happiness, public discontent, and life dissatisfaction (Huppert and Cooper 2014). Social policies have become the vehicle for implementing redistributive programs. Well-being is the main objective of social-public policy in the sense that social, health, educational, economic, domestic, and regional policy issues represent great concern to scholars, government officials, policy makers, and citizens. However, the drivers of well-being and policy issues in the MENA region vary according to the types of government and non-government agencies and actors in each country.

This inquiry has provided an assessment of successful and unsuccessful social policies in the MENA region, which remains one of the most dynamic regions globally, replete with challenges, opportunities, and hopes. Religious charities and private or non-governmental organizations partake in providing social services for meeting the needs of the disabled and low-income citizens. It is essential for policy makers to sustain private sectors as well as to encourage stakeholders to participate in policy processes that can reduce unemployment and create jobs and opportunities for people, particularly the youth in the MENA region. Although significant progress has been made in basic welfare provisions, further development will necessitate greater investment from both the government and the private sector. One of the shortcomings of MENA governments is the adoption of short-term rather than long-term policies. Put differently, the MENA states should move beyond short-term plans that focus on temporary issues such as food and fuel subsidies, to embrace long-term policies focusing on improving human capital as well as on reducing and eliminating inequalities. Governments of the MENA region must implement preventive policies for dealing with problems that threaten the well-being of people before they exist.

The general pattern in the MENA region is that state institutions administer and oversee public policies and impose constraints on civil society organizations and non-government agencies. This statement implies that state institutions are responsible for positive and negative outcomes of social policies. Several scholars have indicated that the conduct of social policy in the MENA region has not been democratic or socially inclusive, and its developmental impact has been minimal or insufficient (el-Aswad 2016; Jawad 2015; Karshenas and Moghadam 2009; Yousef 2004). Countries with austere authoritarian political systems and rigid government regulations tend to have poor social services and fragile civil society organizations. The competent civic state can serve as a powerful means to promote well-being, equality, justice, and peace. Yet, the civic state that does not pay attention to the quality of life and the well-being of its citizens and the public services that oblige them is destined to decline. Policy initiatives that direct weak institutions towards greater equity and legitimacy are needed in order to create multilateral organizations, improve transparency, and increase coordination and effectiveness to achieve the targeted goals of the care and well-being of the people (United Nations Development Programme 2016).

Economic and geopolitical conditions in most MENA countries pose policy challenges for achieving peace, stability, happiness, and quality of life. Examples include the Israeli–Palestinian or Arab–Israeli conflicts, the involvement of global and regional armed forces in Syria's civil war, the Saudi Arabia–Iran conflict, the Saudi-led intervention in Yemen, and the rise of regional and global terrorist groups such as the self-declared Islamic State (IS), previously ISIS or Da'ish (developed from Al-Qa'ida in Iraq), to mention a few. There is increasing recognition of the importance to locate human security at the center of social-public policies in the MENA states. The MENA region, and other regions as well, must adopt clear and practical policies that recommend not only fighting domestic and border-crossing terrorist and violent ideologies and actions but also encourage people to engage in fighting extremism.

Citizens of developing countries are demanding better performance on the part of their governments, and "they are increasingly aware of the costs of poor management and corruption" (World Bank 2005: 1). Promoting integrity and fighting corruption are major challenges to socioeconomic development in the MENA region. Political leaders should go beyond using socioeconomic services to support their short-sighted political interests or legitimacy. Rather, they should serve their countries on equal, democratic, and transparent bases that will, in turn, strengthen their position and dignity as veritable leaders. There is a need for the integration of local, national, regional, and global approaches to enhance well-being and reduce ill-being. Region-building can be achieved through the "process of working toward the integration of a region's social, economic, cultural institutions at all levels of political organization" (Estes 1993: 13).

This study has shown that the drivers, indicators, and outcomes of well-being can guide the policy decisions of governments and those of a broad range of economic, health, and educational institutions/actors such as policy makers, educators, politicians, medical professionals, investors, and shareholders. Serious and well-executed policies regarding strategies for eliminating or reducing poverty and terrorism in the MENA region must be implemented without causing negative outcomes or results that might affect the civil society or prevent decision makers from presenting effective policy options. Citizens should be allowed to play meaningful roles in decision making. And, differences between nations and individuals should be respected (Massam 2002).

Democracy, trustworthy political systems, equality, good health care, quality education, employment, and effective and efficient public services are the greatest demands and needs in the MENA countries. One of the essential policies that needs to be employed is to decentralize government institutions in order to proliferate life satisfaction and help people become happy. More effective policies and initiatives are required to improve health-related well-being by increasing budgets for public health provisions to support hospitals, clinics, and health insurance systems. It is necessary to improve the quality of education at all levels by increasing funding, updating curricula, improving administrative systems, recruiting and training highly qualified instructors, and building reliable educational resources and facilities. The application of advanced technology and innovation in all domains of life must be a priority for public policies in all of the MENA states.

Cooperation and cohesion between the MENA countries is greatly needed. It is worth mentioning that the MENA–Organisation for Economic Co-operation and Development partnership that started in 2005 is a good example of collaboration between countries of the region and economically advanced countries located in other world regions (Organization for Economic Co-operation and Development 2016). But, more efforts are needed to support public and political policies that provide initiatives to solve geopolitical conflicts and political instability across the MENA region. Although domestic reforms remain an important policy issue, regional investment trade and projects will help support the prosperity and stability of the entire region. Projects and initiatives that are shared among MENA countries are vital because these are outstanding investments that can reduce inequality and create jobs as well as ease the flow of wealth and resources. These initiatives could ultimately create the stability and prosperity that the MENA region needs.

The research and policy findings reported in this monograph strongly recommend that states of the MENA region apply well-being research outcomes to articulate significantly enhanced strategic public policies. These initiatives will both promote and sustain the development of public and private policies urgently needed to improve social and cultural endeavors, including health, education, finance, technology, heritage and art, as key drivers toward increasing and advancing quality of life in the region. The lessons learned from the implementation of these initiatives in the MENA almost certainly will give direction to the development of more effective sociocultural policies in other regions of the world that are characterized by high levels of historical, social, political, economic, and even ideological diversity.

References

el-Aswad, el-S. (2016). Political challenges confronting the Islamic World. In H. Tiliouine & R. J. Estes (Eds.), *The state of social progress of Islamic societies: Social, economic, political, and ideological challenges* (pp. 361–377). Cham: Springer International Publishing. https://doi.org/10.1007/978-3-319-24774-8_16.

Estes, R. J. (1993). Toward sustainable development: From theory to praxis. *Social Development Issues, 15*(3), 1–29.

Huppert, F. A., & Cooper, C. L. (2014). *Interventions and policies to enhance wellbeing: A complete reference guide* (Vol. VI). Chichester, West Sussex: Wiley.

Jawad, R. (2015). *Social protection and social policy systems in the MENA region: Emerging trends*. New York: United Nations Department of Economic and Social Affairs.

Karshenas, M., & Moghadam, V. M. (2009) Bringing social policy back in: A look at the Middle East and North Africa. *International Journal of Social Welfare, 18*(1), S52–S61.

Looney, R. E. (2004). Why has globalization eluded the Middle East? *Strategic Insights, 3*(12), 1–14.

Massam, B. H. (2002). Quality of life: Public planning and private living. *Progress in Planning, 58*, 141–227. Retrieved from http://www.tlu.ee/~arro/Happy%20Space%20EKA%202014/quality%20of%20life.pdf.

Organization for Economic Co-operation and Development. (2016). *Middle East and North Africa*. Retrieved from http://www.oecd.org/mena/Active_with_MENA_EN.pdf.

UNESCO. (2012). *Culture: A driver and an enabler of sustainable development: Thematic think piece*. UN System Task Team on the Post-2015 UN Development Agenda. Retrieved from http://www.un.org/millenniumgoals/pdf/Think%20Pieces/2_culture.pdf.

United Nations Development Programme. (2016). *Human development report 2016: Human development for everyone*. New York: United Nations Development Programme. Retrieved from http://hdr.undp.org/sites/default/files/HDR2016_EN_Overview_Web.pdf.

World Bank. (2001). *Cultural heritage and development: A framework for action in the Middle East and North Africa*. Orientations in Development Series. Washington, DC: World Bank. Retrieved from https://openknowledge.worldbank.org/handle/10986/13908.

World Bank. (2005). *Indicators of governance and institutional quality*. Retrieved from http://siteresources.worldbank.org/INTLAWJUSTINST/Resources/IndicatorsGovernanceandInstitutionalQuality.pdf.

World Economic Forum. (2017). *Global competitiveness report* 2016–17. Geneva: World Economic Forum. Retrieved from: http://www3.weforum.org/docs/GCR2016-2017/05FullReport/TheGlobalCompetitivenessReport2016-2017_FINAL.pdf.

Yousef, T. M. (2004). Development, growth and policy reform in the Middle East and North Africa since 1950. *Journal of Economic Perspectives, 18*(3), 91–116.

Index

el-S. el-Aswad, *The Quality of Life and Policy Issues among the Middle East and North African Countries*, Human Well-Being Research and Policy Making,
https://doi.org/10.1007/978-3-030-00326-5

CPSIA information can be obtained
at www.ICGtesting.com
Printed in the USA
LVHW080022061218
599431LV00004B/34/P

9 783030 003258